Kicking the Bucket

From the Common to the Curious, a Look at the Way People Expire

Kim Long and Terry Reim

QUILL

New York

Library of Congress Catalog Card Number: 85-60376

ISBN: 0-688-04712-2

Printed in the United States of America

First Quill Edition

1 2 3 4 5 6 7 8 9 10

RESEARCH AND RESOURCES
Tom Auer
Sally Furgeson
Robert McFarland
Kathleen Cain, Front Range Community College, Westminster,
Colorado
The Denver Public Library
The Boulder Public Library
Norlin Library, University of Colorado, Boulder, Colorado
The Daily Planet Almanac, Boulder, Colorado
The Office for Open Network, Denver, Colorado
National Safety Council
U.S. National Center for Health Statistics
The World Almanac

BOOK DESIGN
Kim Long

TYPESETTING
Argent Typographics, Boulder, Colorado

TECHNICAL SUPPORT
Kicking the Bucket was written, composed, and transmitted to
typesetting equipment on microcomputers from Eagle Computer,
Inc.

This book is respectfully and affectionately dedicated to the authors' fathers, who are still kicking:

Robert I. Long   Jacob V. Reim

"The one thing that makes death distinct from all other diseases and disorders is that everybody gets it."
— Lyall Watson

FOREWORD   6

PREFACE   7

CHAPTER ONE — The Big Picture   8
  □ Death by Definition and the Numbers

CHAPTER TWO — Sick to Death   22
  □ Death by Disease and Medical Misadventure

CHAPTER THREE — Slippery When Wet   56
  □ Death from Accidents

CHAPTER FOUR — On the Move   70
  □ Death from Transportation Mishaps

CHAPTER FIVE — By Their Own Hand   88
  □ Death by Suicide and Self-Destruction

CHAPTER SIX — By Another's Hand   108
  □ Death by Murder and Legal Intervention

CHAPTER SEVEN — On the Battlefield   134
  □ Death by Warfare and Mass Murder

CHAPTER EIGHT — Nature's Way   160
  □ Death from Natural Phenomena

CHAPTER NINE — The Calendar of Death   184
  □ A Daily Dose of Death

APPENDIX   210

INDEX   215

FOREWORD

For centuries, humankind has been preoccupied with life's supreme mystery — death. This preoccupation has been manifested in numerous forms of human behavior, from ancient pagan rites and funerary customs to the science and industry of modern health care.

Yet, recording and compiling information on how people die did not begin until this century; in many underdeveloped parts of the world, reliable vital statistics are still unavailable.

In the U.S., mountains of statistical data for mortality are compiled and disseminated by local, state, and federal agencies each year. Unfortunately, most of us are too overwhelmed by both its quantity and presentation to learn anything from it.

This book serves a useful purpose by selecting and presenting statistical data about death, combined with wise and witty comments by numerous individuals, in an understandable, informative, and interesting manner. Yet, it avoids the often uncontrollable urge to incorrectly analyze, interpret, and explain these statistics.

Many years ago, I studied death in the pathology department of a medical school. It took me another ten years before I realized that I enjoyed two years of performing autopsies because I thought the more I learned about how people die, the more I was protecting myself against this possibility.

Perhaps the readers of this delightful book are similarly motivated. I am aware of no such guarantee, however, on the part of the authors or the publisher. Nonetheless, it does offer entertaining reading about an often unspeakable subject.

As for this old country doctor, I think Diogenes said it best when he told his fellow Athenians 2,400 years ago, "When I die, throw me to the wolves. I'm used to it."

Robert B. McFarland, M.D.

PREFACE

In compiling *Kicking the Bucket*, the authors consulted more than 300 books, periodicals, journals, U.S. government publications, and other manuscripts. We also interviewed numerous individuals from various health care fields who work with death on a day-by-day basis, including medical examiners, physicians, and statisticians.

Statistical data for deaths in the United States is derived exclusively from federal government sources for the year 1980, the most recent year available for all classifications at the time of publication.

The minutiae and anecdotal material are derived primarily from out-of-print publications dated as early as the seventeenth century. The information set in smaller type and located in the outside column of each page is intended to enhance the adjacent text and tabular material.

Although space restrictions necessarily limit the scope of the material presented in this book, we have attempted to include both the most pertinent and the most peculiar fruits of our research. Hopefully, the result is a more animated approach to the reader's understanding of an admittedly lifeless subject.

*"To fear death, gentlemen, is to think
oneself wise when one is not; for it is to
think one knows what one does not know.
No man knows whether death may not
even turn out to be the greatest of blessings
for a human being; and yet people fear it
as if they knew for certain that it is the
greatest of evils."*
— Socrates

Chapter One

THE BIG PICTURE
Death by
Definition and the Numbers

According to Webster's definition, death is "a permanent cessation of all vital functions; the end of life; the cause or occasion of loss of life; the state of being dead." Although civil and legal institutions do not agree on exactly when life ends, most people are able to recognize a corpse without referring to a dictionary. The real mystery lies in the process of dying, and what interaction with the outside world causes a live person to become a dead one. Hopefully, some of the examples, statistics, history, and miscellany presented here will not make this defining process any harder than it already is.

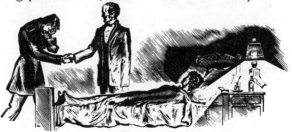

LEGAL DEFINITIONS

The concept of "brain death" emerged in medical circles within the last couple of decades with the advent of transplant surgery and use of respirators. An ad hoc committee of the Harvard Medical School established criteria for describing "irreversible coma":

1) **Unreceptivity and unresponsivity**. The patient shows a total unawareness of externally applied stimuli and inner need, and complete unresponsiveness even when intensely painful stimuli are applied.

2) **No movement or breathing**. All spontaneous muscular movement, spontaneous respiration, and response to stimuli such as pain, touch, sound, or light are absent.

3) **No reflexes**. Among the indications of absent reflex are: fixed, dilated pupils; lack of eye movement even when the head is turned and ice water is placed in the ear; lack of response to noxious stimuli; and generally unelicitable tendon reflexes.

POLLUTION DEATHS

Industrial pollution, including acid rain, causes more than 50,000 fatalities per year in the U.S., according to a Congressional report. The pollution is responsible for generating and aggravating emphysema, pneumonia, and other respiratory diseases. Most of the sources of the pollution involved in this study are coal- and oil-fired power plants in the northeastern states.

Among animals in general, those with larger body sizes have longer life spans; females of most species live longer than males; and spayed females tend to live longer than fertile females.

In 1981, a worker accidentally fell into a brick-making machine in Boulder, Colorado. The fall was unnoticed by other workers, and the machine mixed the man's body into a batch of bricks that were being processed. The bricks from that batch were later buried at a local cemetery.

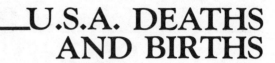

U.S.A. DEATHS AND BIRTHS

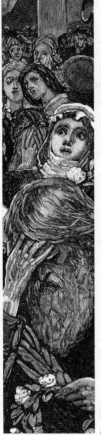

| | BIRTHS | | | |
	Male	Female	Total	Rate (per 100,000)
1955	2,073,719	1,973,576	4,097,000	25.0
1960	2,179,708	2,078,142	4,257,850	23.7
1965	1,927,054	1,833,304	3,760,358	19.4
1970	1,915,378	1,816,008	3,731,386	18.4
1975	1,613,135	1,563,031	3,144,198	14.8
1980	1,853,000	1,760,000	3,613,000	15.9

| | DEATHS | | | |
	Male	Female	Total	Rate (per 100,000)
1955	872,638	656,079	1,528,717	9.3
1960	975,648	736,334	1,711,982	9.5
1965	1,035,200	792,936	1,828,136	9.4
1970	1,078,478	842,553	1,921,031	9.5
1975	1,050,819	842,060	1,892,879	8.9
1980	1,075,000	915,000	1,990,000	8.8

INTERNATIONAL LIFE EXPECTANCIES

Surprisingly enough, the U.S. does not even rank in the top five countries with the longest life expectancies. Sweden, Holland, Norway, Denmark, Canada, France, Japan, and Great Britain all have longer average life expectancies than the U.S.

Among the numerous factors involved in determining life spans is the standard of living, which includes diet, medical care, and health facilities.

HISTORICAL LIFE EXPECTANCIES

"If any question why we died,
Tell them, because our fathers lied."
— Kipling

Below are estimates of the life spans of historic man, based on skeletal remains, gravestones, legal documents, and other factors. These individuals lived to be at least fifteen years of age, therefore, these figures do not reflect infant mortality rates.

NEANDERTHAL MAN	29 years
CRO-MAGNON MAN	32 years
COPPER AGE MAN	36 years
BRONZE AGE MAN	38 years
GREEK & ROMAN MAN	36 years
5TH CENTURY MAN (ENGLISH)	30 years
14TH CENTURY MAN (ENGLISH)	38 years
17TH CENTURY MAN (EUROPEAN)	51 years
18TH CENTURY MAN (EUROPEAN)*	45 years

Epidemics in urban areas are responsible for the reduced life expectancy of eighteenth-century Europeans.

U.S. LIFE EXPECTANCY

	Male	Female	Average
1900	46.3	48.3	47.3
1910	48.4	51.8	50.0
1920	53.6	54.6	54.1
1930	58.1	61.6	59.7
1940	60.8	65.2	62.9
1950	65.6	71.1	68.2
1960	66.6	73.1	69.7
1970	67.1	74.7	70.8
1980	70.0	77.7	73.8

After months of legal struggle, a French women was allowed to wed her dead fiance in 1984. He had been shot to death while on duty as a policeman, and the marriage was performed as the bride held his picture.

During the New York City blackout of November 9, 1965, several people died of heart attacks that were probably related to the situation. Only one person is believed to have died due to an accident directly related to the blackout. A tourist from Florida — attempting to find a way out of his hotel — walked into an open elevator shaft and fell to his death.

HOW LONG DO YOU HAVE TO LIVE?

There have been nine accidental deaths at Disneyland since it opened in 1955. On the average, there are seven deaths per year at amusement parks in the U.S.

AVERAGE LIFETIME IN THE U.S. (1980)

Age Interval	Number Of Living	Average Life Expectancy
0-1	100,000	73.6
1-5	98,743	73.6
5-10	98,486	69.8
10-15	98,323	64.9
15-20	98,174	60.0
20-25	97,676	55.3
25-30	97,011	50.6
30-35	96,353	45.9
35-40	95,649	41.3
40-45	94,797	36.6
45-50	93,469	32.1
50-55	91,380	27.8
55-60	88,126	23.7
60-65	83,324	19.9
65-70	76,545	16.4
70-75	67,640	13.3
75-80	56,355	10.4
80-85	41,431	8.2
85 & over	26,395	6.5

A study of Italian duels between 1880 and 1890 puts the total number of duels at 2,760, with fifty fatalities. The involved parties consisted of military men (30 percent), editors (29 percent), lawyers (12 percent), and other occupations (29 percent). There are no figures given for which profession got the worst of it.

OLD AND COLD

It is estimated that about 25,000 elderly people die from hypothermia (over exposure to the cold) each year in the U.S. While some of these deaths are undoubtedly attributable to a lack of heat in the home, many result from the victims' weakened condition from illness and old age, and from a lack of information about how to stay warm. Also, some prescription drugs (including Valium and the phenothiazines) can increase vulnerability to hypothermia. Most victims of the cold live where the temperature is between 30 and 50 degrees Fahrenheit.

AUTOPSIES

"So we must part, my body, you and I
Who've spent so many pleasant years together.
'Tis sorry work to lose your company
Who clove to me so close."
— Cosmo Monkhouse

In 1979, all states in the U.S. required that death certificates show whether an autopsy had been performed. Of a total 1,913,841 deaths during that year, autopsies were ordered in 294,182 cases, making the 1979 autopsy rate 15.4 percent.

The percentage of autopsies has decreased steadily over the past twenty-five years, primarily because fewer autopsies have been performed on deaths attributed to the three major causes of death: heart disease, cancer, and stroke. These three causes account for two-thirds of the total deaths in the U.S. In 1979, autopsies were performed on only 9.3 percent of such victims.

On the other hand, the percentage of autopsies performed in three other categories — homicide, suicide, and accidents — has steadily increased over the past twenty-five years. Homicide autopsies went from 60.16 percent in 1958 to 93.2 percent in 1979. Suicide autopsies increased from 21.7 percent to 45.2 percent during the same period. The accidental

Captain James Cook, explorer, was killed in 1779 by Hawaiian natives, with whom he had had a disagreement. He was stabbed and drowned, and his body rendered into pieces. Parts of Cook — his scalp, bare bones, and both hands preserved in salt — were returned to his crew, who buried the remains at sea.

In Plymouth, England, a legal battle was being fought in 1984 over the right of a local artist to embalm the dead body of a friend and keep it as a memento.

A private study — conducted by the mother of a college student accidentally killed during a fraternity hazing — lists sixty-five fatalities known to have been related to hazing practices on U.S. campuses.

death autopsy figures rose from 26.8 percent to 42.6 percent. While these causes of death represented only 8 percent of all deaths, autopsies were conducted on an average of 50.4 percent of them.

The expense involved in a complete autopsy has increased substantially over the past twenty-five years, and government agencies are more reluctant to incur this cost. If a family desires an autopsy that has been deemed unnecessary, they must bear the financial burden of the procedure which can cost thousands of dollars.

A waterbed fatality was reported in California in 1983. The owner of the bed had fallen asleep while waiting for the bed to fill with water; he suffocated when the fluid-filled mattress rolled over on him.

MORBID MEMORIES

Reflections of Dr. Hal Wagner
Chief Pathologist,
Cook County, Illinois 1958-1964

"You can assume that one percent of the population dies every year. Of this number, upwards of 500,000 will become coroner's cases. Those of us who work in this field expect a certain number of murders in an area, based on how tightly packed people are — a specific density per square mile.

"Suicides are not really a matter of opinion with coroners, but I was always willing to give the dead guy the benefit of the doubt."

"I know from experience that people who slit their wrists don't just do it in one stroke. They make initial attempts and these cuts are called 'hesitation marks.' You look for these when suicide is in question.

"Can you get away with murder? I doubt it. Someone can't know for sure that a coroner won't be called in. I remember a case that was signed out and then two days later, some character in Fort Wayne had a fit of conscience and called the cops to say he'd shot his girlfriend. The body wasn't buried, so I was called in. I went and took a look and found a bullet wound under her armpit that went all the way through. This had been signed out as a cardiac arrest.

"The purpose of a coroner is not to find murders. That's only a small adjunct to what they do. An autopsy is often done on persons under forty. If someone is under forty, I don't believe he should die a natural death, so I'll contact his doctor, anyone I can, to find out if the dead person had an illness, etc. If I can't find anything out, I'll take twenty minutes and take a look.

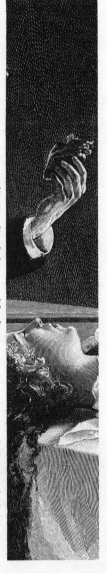

"The rule in suicide is: if an individual is doing what he normally does and he ends up dead — say, of an overdose — this is probably an accident.

"People who are drunk generally do not commit suicide. I believe that being drunk makes a person incapable of making the decision to end his own life.

"In the first part of the 19th century, there was a big scandal. There was a fee given to funeral directors for burying indigent children. As it turned out, some funeral directors were stealing kids, killing them, and getting the fee. This is what led to the death certificate. In this country now, a funeral director can't bury anybody without a death certificate."

_____PRESIDENTIAL DEATH FACTS

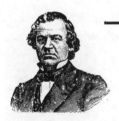

"The sense of death is most in apprehension,
And the poor beetle that we tread upon
In corporal sufferance finds a pang as great
As when a giant dies."
— Shakespeare

The first Vice President to die in office was George Clinton, who died on April 20, 1812, in Washington, D.C.

☐ Sixteen lived to be at least seventy years old.

☐ Thirty-one died from natural causes; four were assassinated.

☐ Eight died while holding office.

☐ Three died on July 4; John Adams and Thomas Jefferson died on the same day, July 4, 1826.

☐ Seven died in the month of July.

☐ The average life span for Presidents is sixty-nine years and ninety-five days.

☐ No President has ever died in the month of May.

☐ Two Democrats and four Republicans have died in office; both Presidents in the Whig party died in office.

William Rufus De Vane King, thirteenth Vice President of the U.S., died of tuberculosis in 1853 — although alcoholism probably was a contributing factor. In his last political campaign, he had been labelled "a hero of many a well-fought bottle." At the time of inauguration, he was in Havana, Cuba, too sick to return to Washington.

_____VICE PRESIDENTIAL DEATH FACTS

☐ Four Vice Presidents died in office.

☐ Eight died in November.

☐ The average life span for Vice Presidents is seventy-one years and 251 days.

☐ Twenty-one lived to be at least seventy years old.

_____BIORHYTHMS AND DEATH

"Around, around the sun we go:
The moon goes round the earth.
We do not die of death:
We die of vertigo."
— Archibald Macleish

The theory of biorhythms, as it is now known, was originally the brainchild of a German doctor named Wilhelm Fliess. Dr. Fliess was a noted medical specialist in the late 1800s, but he achieved fame and popularity in his lifetime for another theory, one suggesting that there was a direct connection between a person's sexual organs and his or her nose. Much of his research involved studying and manipulating noses in a therapeutic attempt to overcome various physical problems. One of his biggest fans was Sigmund Freud, who was introduced by Dr. Fliess to the ultimate nasal treatment, cocaine.

Dr. Fliess was also a student of cycles, and he observed what he believed to be direct correlations between the time a person was born and how he interacted with the world. This theory represented the beginning of biorhythms, but was refined and adapted by many other researchers before it became widely accepted. Dr. Fliess received little support for this idea, and was stuck with the fame of his nasal cures.

Biorhythms are currently understood to be composed of three separate cycles which begin at the moment a person is born. These cycles — emotional, intellectual, and physical — alternate between high and low phases on different schedules. The emotional cycle runs for twenty-

James Schoolcraft Sherman, the twenty-seventh Vice President of the U.S., died in 1912 of uremic poisoning only a few days before the election for his and Taft's second term. No replacement was offered by the party, and 3,484,980 people cast their votes for a dead man on election day.

During the construction of the original London Bridge over the Thames River, at least 250 workers are known to have died in the thirty-three years it took to complete the structure.

eight days, the intellectual cycle for thirty-three days, and the physical cycle for twenty-three days. Any time a cycle changes from high to low or from low to high, a critical period exists.

During a critical period, which is thought to last for only a day, a dangerous potential prevails. At this time, there is supposedly a greater tendency for accidents to happen and a greater potential for death. Studies have been done to determine if, as expected, more people die during critical periods than at other times. Unfortunately, there seems to be no clear consensus from the results.

An investigation into transportation accident statistics in 1939 showed that of 300 recorded deaths, 197 had occurred on critical days. This is 65 percent of the total, which is much larger than a random selection would show. On the other hand, a 1977 study of 506 traffic accidents with fatalities involved, revealed no correlation with biorhythms, nor did several studies of aviation accidents.

There have been thirty-five presidential deaths in the United States. An examination of the times of death of these indicated that ten died on critical days (eight when one cycle was critical, and two when more than one cycle was critical at the same time). A mathematical model for these individuals would produce virtually the same results as chance. One interesting detail: William McKinley was shot on a non-critical day but died several days later, when a critical period was in effect.

Famous deaths on critical days:
☐ Marilyn Monroe (drug overdose)
☐ Janis Joplin (drug overdose)
☐ George Armstrong Custer (Indian problems)
☐ Judy Garland (drug overdose)
☐ Clark Gable (heart attack)

A Swedish historian known as Rudbeck was said to have died from grief after losing a major book on the history of Sweden (which he had just completed) in a fire.

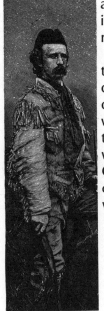

DEATH BY STARVATION

"Out of the chill and the shadow,
Into the thrill and the shrine;
Out of the dearth and the famine,
Into the fullness divine."
— Margaret E. Sangster

Death by starvation can take about ten weeks for an adult human male. Famine is the starvation of a larger proportion of the population over a wide geographical area. When severe enough and widespread enough, famine can cause millions of deaths within a period of a year or two.

Unlike other natural calamities, famine is rarely a sudden emergency. It occurs from a gradual dwindling of the food supply, usually caused by weather abnormalities such as drought, early or late frost, massive rains, and flooding, which destroy crops. Other less common causes of famine are insect infestations and wars. Some armies have deliberately destroyed or confiscated harvests on a massive scale, leaving the civilian population to starve.

Famine was probably unknown before the Neolithic revolution transformed humans from nomadic hunters to "stationary" farmers, dependent on weather conditions for crop cultivation and livestock care. Thereafter, famine was probably responsible for more deaths among all civilizations than anything else but disease (especially plagues). Although Europe has been less prone to famine than Asia, between 0 and 1800 A.D., famines occurred in Europe approximately one year out of every five, causing untold suffering and the deaths of millions.

In Asia, especially India and China, loss of life

During the Mongol invasion in the thirteenth century, warriors were held responsible for measured quotas of dead civilians; the count was kept with severed ears. In the city of Merv (Persia), over 700,000 people were killed in the month of February, 1221.

In July, 1981, the first known fatality caused by a robot occurred in a Japanese factory, when Kenji Urada, a maintenance worker, was accidentally killed by an automated assembly machine.

On the average, about ten football players die every year in the U.S., at all levels of competition, from sandlot to professional. Most of these deaths, about 60 percent, result from head injuries. This average was higher — more than thirty deaths a year — until the late 1960s.

In a comprehensive study of Herman Melville's works, a researcher discovered that in eleven novels there were 1,802 items relating to death, including fatalities, deaths in nature, and general references to death.

from famine historically has been astronomical. During the first half of the nineteenth century, 45 million people starved to death in China alone; in the previous half-century in India, an estimated 35 million people perished from famine.

Severe and prolonged famines have inevitably been accompanied by cannibalism, regardless of political and religious abhorrence. Children were usually the primary victims of this practice, often eaten by their parents.

Although twentieth-century technology has improved agricultural efficiency and production, famine, starvation, and hunger are by no means relics of the past. Thousands still die annually from starvation in the underdeveloped parts of the world, especially on the African continent.

International relief organizations have significantly affected starvation mortality in the world, but political conflicts, droughts, and monoculture cash-crop farming have allowed chronic starvation, hunger, and malnutrition to remain pervasive throughout much of the world.

Throughout this brief survey of starvation, references to mortality are based only upon deaths directly attributable to starvation.

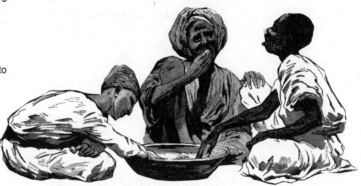

___MAJOR FAMINES OF THE TWENTIETH CENTURY

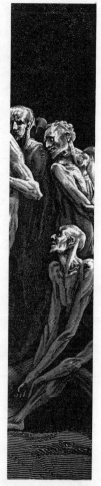

- ☐ **India**: 1899-1901 — One million perish in famine.
- ☐ **China**: 1911 — Millions perish from starvation.
- ☐ **Russia**: 1911 — Devastating famine kills millions.
- ☐ **Armenia**: 1916 — Tens of thousands starve to death.
- ☐ **China**: 1928 — About 3 million perish of starvation over a three-year period.
- ☐ **USSR**: 1932-1934 — Famine devastates new social order; 5 million starve to death.
- ☐ **China**: 1936 — Famine caused by drought; 5 million starve to death in the western part of the country.
- ☐ **India**: 1943 — Millions die in famine during World War II.
- ☐ **China**: 1943 — In Kwang Tung Province, one million starve to death. The sale of children becomes common.
- ☐ **USSR**: 1947 — Tens of thousands of peasants starve to death in the wake of grain exports (not reported until 1963).
- ☐ **Nigeria**: 1968 — Death toll estimates of severe famine range from 800,000 to millions, during a three-month period.
- ☐ **Africa** and **India**: 1973-1974 — Mass starvation; 200,000 perish.
- ☐ **Central Africa**: 1980-present — The first live television coverage of a major famine; millions of TV viewers witness the deaths of thousands in prime time.

Mass poisoning by mercury killed more than 450 people in Iraq in 1971.

"In the long run . . . we are all dead."
— J. Maynard Keynes

Chapter Two

SICK TO DEATH
Death by
Disease and Medical Misadventure

Throughout history, disease has killed more people worldwide than any other cause. In fact, nothing else even comes close. But of all diseases, one stands out as the leading killer throughout history — malaria. Malaria still kills between a million and a million-and-a-half people annually, and is increasing once again.

Malaria is carried by 24 of the 200 species of Anopheles mosquito which breeds on the surface of still waters. These mosquitoes are inhabited by a parasitic organism, the one-celled malaria plasmodia, which spends half its life in mosquitoes and the other half in the blood stream of mammals. These lethal parasites have invaded 70 percent of the world's land masses and have caused more suffering and death to the human race than anything else in history.

Malaria is an ancient disease. Records of malaria go back 3,500 years; Hippocrates noted its occurrence as "intermittent fevers" long associated with swamps and the heat of summer. Unlike many other diseases, it can kill immediately or can subside and recur chronically until the victim eventually succumbs to the debilitating effects of continual relapses.

Alexander the Great almost certainly died of malaria, and Julius Caesar suffered from the disease. For generations, Rome was so plagued by this scourge it was called "the pestilential city."

Before the time of Columbus, malaria had spread from its breeding ground in the Mediterranean throughout Europe, and as far north as Denmark. In England, where it was called "the ague," it sometimes raged so fiercely that there were not enough able-bodied people to harvest the crops, which in turn led to famine.

There is no known vaccine for malaria. In the late 1950s, international efforts to eliminate the breeding grounds of mosquitoes with insecticides made a significant impact on the death rate and saved an estimated 400 million from the disease. But premature discontinuance of these programs, along with acquired resistance to DDT by the mosquitoes, has resulted in a resurgence of the disease, an estimated 2.3-fold increase in its prevalence.

The most destructive disease in history is malaria. Over a million-and-a-half people die from malaria every year, and it is found in more than 70 percent of the world's land masses.

Ivan the Terrible, Czar of Russia, died in 1584 from an unknown ailment that caused him "grievously to swell in the cods."

PARASITIC ILLNESSES

"Who, then, is free? The wise man who can command his passions, who fears not want, nor death, nor chains . . ."
— Horace

More than a billion people worldwide suffer from some form of parasitic illness. Although most apparent in underdeveloped areas, infestations occur nearly everywhere. Roundworm is the most common parasite, affecting almost a billion people. These worms thrive in the intestines of people as well as in the intestines of pigs and other domestic animals. While roundworm is the most prevalent of parasitic diseases, malaria is the most deadly. The sporozoan parasites that cause malaria affect some 800 million people and kill 1.2 million every year.

Although they are widespread, parasitic diseases have not generated much funding for research. For instance, the U.S. government spends less than $1 million annually on hookworm research, even though this parasite infects 900 million people. On the other hand, the U.S. government spends $815 million on research of cancer, a disease that affects ten million people.

Thalidomide, a sedative that was prescribed to thousands of pregnant mothers in the early 1960s in many different countries, was responsible for the birth of hundreds of deformed babies and between 3,000 and 5,000 deaths.

PARASITIC ILLNESSES WORLDWIDE

Disease	Infected (in millions)	Fatalities per Year (in thousands)
Malaria	800	1,200
Bilharziasis	200	500-1,000
— South American	12	60
Hookworm	900	50-60
Onchocerciasis	30	20-50
Amebiasis	400	30
Roundworm	1,000	20
Leishmaniasis	12	5
Trypanosomiasis — African	1	5
Trichuriasis	500	Low
Filariasis	250	Low
Giardiasis	200	Very Low

DEAD HEADHUNTERS

In one of the most bizarre medical mysteries known to science, hundreds of primitive tribesmen who lived in the eastern highlands of New Guinea were discovered to be dropping dead of an unknown disease in the 1950s. After years of research and tests, the mystery of this disease — called Kuru — was solved, but a cure has never been found.

The deaths were puzzling because they could not be attributed to any known organism, contagious behavior, or local food source. Most of those affected were female adults, but of the 25 percent that were children, equal numbers of males and females were stricken. In some areas, the disease had infected 10 percent of the local population, and was responsible for 50 percent of all of the deaths.

The mystery was finally solved when it was discovered that the practice of cannibalism had not entirely disappeared as had been previously reported. An established tradition of eating the brains of deceased relatives was continuing in secret. As part of this mourning ritual, women and children were responsible for preparing the brain of the dead person for eating, and thus were exposed to much more of this tissue than were the adult men. The final part of the riddle was solved when it was proven that the mysterious virus that was causing the deaths could only be transmitted through contact with the body tissue where it thrived — the brain.

The difficult and unique medical detective work that helped solve the riddle of this obscure fatal virus led to a Nobel Prize in 1976 to Dr. Carleton

The will of Mrs. Martin Van Butchell, who died in 1775, stated that her husband could control her money only as long as her body remained above the ground — he paid an anatomist to find a way to preserve her body, which was then put on display, and was thought to be the beginning of modern embalming practices.

Catheters are often used for patients with bladder problems in health-care institutions — at least 7.5 million are inserted each year in the U.S. Recent studies indicate that as many as 56,000 patients may die every year from infections related to these catheters. Although the catheters are suspected to be the cause of these fatalities, medical researchers have yet to isolate the specific relationship and develop a cure.

Public records from 1860 report that a baby in Bellevue Hospital in New York City was killed by rats, which were a common pest in hospitals of that era.

Gajdusek, who was in charge of the research. The natives "cured" themselves, as their cannibalistic mourning rituals gradually disappeared.

____HEART DISEASE WORLDWIDE

"To fear love is to fear life, and those who fear life are already three parts dead."
— Bertrand Russell

In the United States, and in most of the advanced countries of the world, CVD is the number one cause of death by an overwhelming margin. About half of all deaths in the U.S. — almost a million annually — are attributed to CVD.

In most countries (the U.S. excluded), women are more likely to die of heart disease than men, except for the 45-64 age group, where the risk is greater for men worldwide. For both sexes, the risk of death from heart disease is greatest in the plus 65 age group.

The following rankings seem to confirm the widely held notion that there is a causal relation between heart disease and lifestyle. Urbanites seem more prone to this malady than individuals who populate rural environs. There appears to be overwhelming evidence that heart disease is indeed a malady of civilization. The highest ranking non-Western non-caucasian nation — the Philippines — ranks thirty-seventh out of forty-five selected countries, representing the highest to lowest mortality rates from heart disease worldwide for 1980.

HEART DISEASE WORLDWIDE

DEADLIEST COUNTRIES	DEATH RATE (per 100,000)
Hungary	685.2
Scotland	662.3
Sweden	583.6
LEAST DEADLY COUNTRIES	
Syria	53.4
Guatemala	48.4
Thailand	25.3

(The U.S. ranks eleventh worldwide: 436.4 deaths per 100,000 population.)

A European medical study indicated that more people die natural deaths in Western Europe from December through February than any other time of the year, with the opposite being the case from July through August, when the fewest die.

While the death rate between the top and bottom countries from this list represents a remarkable disparity (685.2 for Hungary compared to 25.3 for Thailand), citizens of countries in the lower category are not as fortunate as it might initially appear.

As it turns out, life expectancy for these same nations would generally correspond to the above rankings. Since most heart disease mortalities occur among the elderly, especially in the above-65 age group, a relatively small number of people will die of heart disease if most of the population tends to die of other causes at an earlier age. Just such a circumstance is reflected here.

When embalming was first becoming acceptable, some embalmers took corpses on exhibition tours of barbershops, country fairs, and public halls in order to solicit new business.

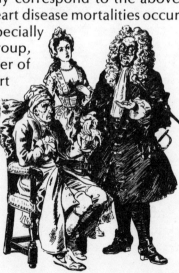

THE U.S.A.'S BIGGEST KILLER

In a study of drug reactions in Great Britain for a seven-year-period up to 1971, it was discovered that there were 592 deaths from anti-inflammatory analgesics, 332 deaths from oral contraceptives, 217 deaths from phenyl-butazone (for rheumatism and arthritis), and 102 deaths from chlorpromazine.

"He who pretends to look on death without fear lies. All men are afraid of dying, this is the great law of sentient beings, without which the entire human species would soon be destroyed."
— Jean-Jacques Rousseau

Of the almost two million people who die in the U.S. every year, half die of "heart disease." More accurately referred to as cardiovascular disease (CVD), it is responsible for almost a million deaths annually in the U.S. — as many as all other causes combined.

Arteriosclerosis, an accumulation of fatty deposits within the arteries, is regarded as the major underlying cause of CVD. This condition can be attributed to high cholesterol levels, smoking, and high blood pressure.

Cardiovascular diseases are divided into five categories: heart attack, stroke, high blood pressure, rheumatic heart disease, and coronary heart disease. Stroke, however, is usually listed separately as the third leading cause of death. At least 42,750,000 Americans have one or more forms of heart or blood vessel disease.

A United Nations report from 1969 estimated the total fatalities caused by exposure to radiation from nuclear weapons testing (all tests worldwide, from the first test to 1969). Their estimate: 35,040 to 84,540.

MICROWAVE PARANOIA

Despite the ominous warnings found in most public establishments that use microwave ovens, no known human fatalities have resulted from this man-made radiation. The warnings, which are not required by law, apparently date back to a Navy-sponsored test with laboratory monkeys. In February of 1970, information was released that a single monkey had died after several hours of exposure to microwave radiation. This, plus evidence that heavy microwave radiation can damage the eyes, provided ammunition for several national columnists, who started a wave of public concern.

Robert Wadlow, the tallest man in the world, died in 1940 at the age of twenty-two from a severe infection caused by the braces he wore to help him stand up. He was eight-feet, eleven-inches tall and weighed 491 pounds at the time of his death.

HEARTLAND OF AMERICA

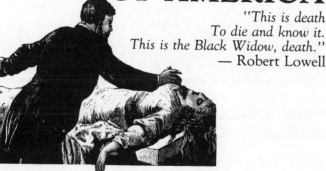

"This is death
To die and know it.
This is the Black Widow, death."
— Robert Lowell

In 1980, 980,100 deaths occurred in the U.S. from some form of CVD, constituting a death rate of 436.4 per 100,000 nationally. Regionally, there is a significant variation in death rates. The Rocky Mountain region exhibited the lowest death rate at 232.9, and the Middle Atlantic region had the highest death rate from CVD in 1980, with 421.1.

In the state-by-state breakdown, Pennsylvania ranks highest for CVD mortalities, with a 1980 rate of 428.4; New York is a close second at 426.3; and Rhode Island comes in third at 404.5. Alaska is the state with the lowest death rate, an incredible 91.3; New Mexico is next lowest at 177.5, almost twice the

Bloodletting, once used by physicians as a popular "catch-all" cure, was responsible for many untimely deaths. Charles II of England was one of these, expiring in 1685 the day after sixteen ounces of his blood was removed by royal doctors in an attempt to treat an unknown illness.

In 1937, a medicine for anti-bacterial use was distributed by Massengill & Company. In order to get the active ingredient to dissolve, it was mixed with diethylene glycol, also used in anti-freeze solutions for automobiles. Before the error could be corrected, there were at least seventy-three deaths related to use of this product, and the chemist responsible for mixing the formula committed suicide.

rate of Alaska. These are the only two states with a CVD death rate for 1980 lower than 200.

—————HEART HISTORY

In 1900, only one-fifth of all deaths in the U.S. were attributed to CVD. By the time World War I began, CVD was the leading cause of death and has remained so ever since, except for 1918, when a worldwide flu epidemic eclipsed it in U.S. mortalities. Between 1900 and 1980, the death rate for heart disease almost doubled in the U.S. — from 169.2 to 336.0. By 1925, one-third of all deaths in the U.S. were caused by heart disease; by 1960, CVD accounted for half of all deaths.

——————————HEART BREAKDOWN

"Many men would take the death-sentence
without a whimper to escape the life-
sentence which fate carries in her other hand."
— T. E. Lawrence

Cardiovascular Disease is classified into five major categories:

☐ **HEART ATTACK**. Arteriosclerosis causes a narrowing of the arteries supplying the heart muscle with oxygen and food until parts of the heart die and it stops pumping. When a blood clot forms in the artery, doctors call it a coronary thrombosis, coronary occlusion, or myocardial infarction. Angina pectoris occurs when narrowed arteries cannot deliver sufficient oxygen to the heart muscle, thus causing chest pains in the victim. About 1,500,000 people will have a heart attack this year, of which 559,000 will not survive. Four-and-a-half million people who have a history of heart attacks or angina are alive today.

☐ **HIGH BLOOD PRESSURE**. Although the causes are unknown, high blood pressure is a condition where the pressure of the circulatory system is great enough to create a strain on the heart and blood vessels. Sometimes this enlarges the heart. More than 31,800 deaths were caused by high blood pressure in 1981. An estimated 37 million Americans suffer from this affliction.

☐ **STROKE**. When a blood clot occurs in an artery of the brain, or when a vessel in the brain ruptures, a stroke occurs. Portions of the brain are usually damaged, and if death does not result, paralysis, or other dysfunction can debilitate the victim for the rest of his life. Strokes caused by clots are called cerebral thrombosis. Strokes affect a total of half-a-million Americans and cause about 164,000 deaths every year. There are 2 million surviving stroke victims. Stroke, (cerebrovascular disease) is the third leading cause of death in the U.S.; figures for stroke deaths are not included in death rate and mortalities for CVD.

☐ **RHEUMATIC HEART DISEASE**. This is a condition where the heart's valves are damaged by strepto-coccal infection. If untreated, rheumatic fever can occur. About 7,700 deaths are attributed to this cause annually. More than 2 million victims of this affliction are alive today.

☐ **CONGENITAL HEART DISEASE**. About 25,000 babies are born with heart abnormalities every year and about 6,500 die annually from these abnormalities. Almost half-a-million are afflicted but alive today.

The number one cause of death in the U.S. and most of the countries of the world is heart disease.

Dr. Charles Drew, the doctor responsible for developing plasma, died in 1950 from injuries suffered in an automobile crash. An unsubstantiated story was circulated at the time claiming he was refused admission to a local hospital after the accident because he was black, and subsequently died from lack of blood.

____HEART DEATHS BY AGE AND SEX

The drug Clofibrate, was introduced in 1963 for the reduction of cholesterol levels and prevention of heart attacks. In an international test over many years, it was shown that although the drug apparently reduced the numbers of non-fatal heart attacks, the number of fatal heart attacks increased.

Heart disease is primarily an affliction of the old; it accounts for the vast majority of deaths among people older than forty-five. As life expectancy increased during this century from the elimination of infectious diseases, the incidence of heart disease showed a similar increase. In the old days many people didn't live long enough to die of heart disease.

UNITED STATES DEATH RATES PER 100,000

	Male	Female
15-24	3.7	2.1
25-44	34.6	11.9
45-64	505.3	177.3
65 and over	2,778.6	2,027.5
All Ages	368.6	305.1

Male And Female
All Ages   336.0

____STROKING OUT

Ibuprofen, a drug prescribed for reducing inflammation, can be fatal to individuals who have a sensitivity to its activity, but there is no way to detect this sensitivity until an attack occurs. It is currently available in the U.S.

Stroke is a form of cardiovascular disease that effects the blood vessels carrying food and oxygen to the brain. Referred to as cerebrovascular disease, stroke is the third leading cause of death in the U.S. Figures for 1980 listed stroke deaths at 170,200, giving it a mortality rate of 75.1.

Like other cardiovascular diseases, the contributing factors to stroke include obesity, lack of exercise, smoking, high cholesterol diet, and stress. A stroke victim who survives is often faced with lifelong impairment of physical and/or mental capabilities. Such brain damage will affect the opposite side of the body.

Stroke has numerous forms, some of the more common of which include:

☐ **CEREBRAL THROMBOSIS**. This common form of stroke occurs when a clot forms inside a cerebral blood vessel, usually due to artherosclerosis.

☐ **CEREBRAL EMBOLISM**. A wandering clot finally lodges in an artery leading to the brain.

☐ **CEREBROVASCULAR OCCLUSION**. This occurs whenever a clot plugs a cerebral artery as in both of the above instances.

☐ **CEREBRAL HEMORRHAGE**. This form is the bursting of a defective artery or aneurysm, which floods surrounding brain tissue with blood.

At the turn of the century in the U.S., influenza and pneumonia were the leading causes of death. In 1918, when an epidemic of flu swept through the country, more than half-a-million died.

INFLUENZA AND PNEUMONIA

"Dying is not everything: you have to die in time."
— Jean-Paul Sartre

Modern standards of classifying the causes of death rank influenza and pneumonia together as the fourth leading cause of death among twenty-seven major classifications. Influenza/pneumonia have been responsible for about 50,000 deaths annually for the past few years, claiming about the same number of fatalities as auto accidents and chronic pulmonary obstructions. The latest U.S. figures (1980) show an influenza/pneumonia death rate of 24.1 per 100,000 population.

In 1900, influenza and pneumonia were the leading causes of death in the U.S. The death rate then for these two diseases was 202.2 per 100,000

Thomas Jefferson, third President of the U.S., died in 1826 from diarrhea. James Knox Polk, eleventh President of the U.S., died in 1849 from the same cause.

DPX, or dextro-propoxyphene — sometimes marketed in the U.S. as Darvon — is considered by some experts to be the most deadly drug available by prescription. Only two or three times the normal doses can be fatal, and death is possible in as little as thirty minutes.

Estimates of deaths in the U.S. from reactions to prescribed drugs range from 10,000 to 130,000 per year.

A statistical study from the 1950s in the U.S. showed that there was a higher death rate for widows, widowers, and divorcees than among single and married persons of the same age group.

population. In 1918, a global flu epidemic struck, followed by a secondary wave of pneumonia. Of an estimated 20 million Americans who contracted the influenza, more than half-a-million died, and the mortality rate rose to 584.5.

While the death toll directly attributable to influenza/pneumonia has been reduced to one-tenth of the 1900 statistics, these two illnesses — influenza especially — are often underlying factors in the deaths of people who suffer from other chronic diseases or conditions.

Mortality from pneumonia and the flu is highly seasonal. More than three times as many deaths occur in the peak months of January and February than in the low month of August. This seasonal pattern is also apparent in secondary illness and disability caused by flu and pneumonia.

The differences in mortality rates for various age groups is also dramatic: those at the extremes of life have proven most susceptible to the fatal effects of the two illnesses. Infants under one year of age showed the highest mortality rate (261 per 100,000 in 1958) and the above-80 age group had a mortality rate of more than 750 for the same year.

There is also a marked gender and race difference in the mortality rates. In 1900, the mortality rate for men was slightly greater than that for women. Since that time, women appear to have benefited more from advances in medicine. For example, in 1958, the mortality rate among all age groups and all geographical areas and races was 59 percent higher for males than females. Listings by race show that more than twice as many non-whites as whites died of flu or pneumonia that year. The male/female ratio within these two groups, however, remained essentially the same. For both whites and non-whites, about 60 percent of the total deaths were male.

Climate and geography seem to have little effect on mortality from flu and pneumonia. However, occupation does seem to matter. Higher than average pneumonia death rates have been observed among certain professions, such as welding, mining, and any profession involving exposure to dusts, gasses, excessive fatigue, or extremes of temperature. Additionally, alcoholics and those from the lower socio-economic brackets show an above average death rate from pneumonia.

_____SCHOOL DAZE

In 1982, an outbreak of meningitis occurred in a Texas elementary school. Of the seven students who contracted the disease, one died. A mini-epidemic of this disease is rare, and medical experts who studied the case theorized that because only girls were victims, the contagion resulted from the girls sitting too close together in a classroom. Apparently the teacher had placed the girls and boys on opposite sides of the room and, because there were more girls than boys, the extra space between the boys provided protection that the girls did not have.

Only one or two berries from the mistletoe plant are needed to cause death in a child. The lethal dose of holly berries for children is twenty to thirty.

After undergoing several months of continuing exorcism by a Roman Catholic priest, Anneliese Michel, a West German college student, died in 1976 at the age of twenty-three from malnutrition and dehydration. As a result of her death, the Church added a requirement that a doctor always be present during exorcisms.

_____TUBERCULOSIS

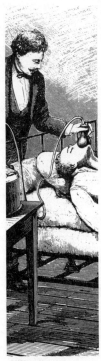

"Nothing that is extreme is evil. Death comes to you? It would be dreadful could it remain with you; but of necessity either it does not arrive or else it departs."
— Seneca

At the turn of the twentieth century, tuberculosis (TB) claimed second place among the leading causes of death in the U.S. The TB mortality rate in 1900 was 199 per 100,000 population, second only to influenza/pneumonia with a death rate of 202.2.

Since that time, however, the mortality rate for TB has declined consistently and dramatically. In 1980, the tuberculosis death toll totaled only 2,000, resulting in a TB mortality rate for that year of 0.9.

Today, the elderly account for most of the TB fatalities, with elderly male deaths being slightly more prevalent than elderly female deaths. Otherwise, the disease seems to strike both sexes in equal proportion.

About one-third of all deaths from automobile accidents occur in ambulances after the wrecks and in hospital emergency rooms within a few minutes of the arrival of the victims.

Among the elderly, racial differences appear to have little effect on mortality rates. However, mortality rates for younger ages show that non-whites perish from this disease at three times the rate of whites. Contraction of and death from TB usually reflect differences in socio-economic backgrounds: the victims are primarily from the lower end of the economic spectrum.

There is also a geographical factor in TB prevalence, caused in these times primarily by socio-economic and geographical divisions. As could be expected, high mortality rates exist in areas that attract a high number of TB patients for treatment.

CANCER PROGNOSIS

"Alone of gods Death has no love for gifts,
Libation helps you not, nor sacrifice.
He has no altar, and he hears no hymns;
From him alone Persuasion stands apart."
— Aeschylus

Washington, D.C., has the highest fatality rate from cancer in the U.S., and Alaska has the lowest rate.

Cancer, a word that strikes fear in the stoutest of hearts, is losing some of its panic-inspiring qualities with every passing year. In 1984, almost 870,000 Americans were diagnosed as having cancer. About 326,000 of them, or 39 percent, will survive for five years or more. This "observed" survival rate is double the cancer survival rate of fifty years ago. According to the American Cancer Society, of the 544,000 who will not survive this year, an additional 148,000 could have been saved by earlier diagnosis and prompt treatment. With early detection, many cancers can be cured by X-rays, radioactive substances, chemicals, hormones, or immuno-therapy.

The Joseph Family Disease is confined to the members of a single family, and has been traced to the arrival of a Portuguese sailor in California in 1845. Joseph family members who contract the disease suffer from a degeneration of the nervous system that leads to death.

Through the 1960s and early 1970s, the cancer patient's chances of survival remained one-in-three. Recent medical developments in diagnostic techniques and sophisticated treatment procedures have increased a patient's chances to three-in-eight, or, again, 39 percent. This means that an additional 40,000 Americans — who, fifteen years ago, would have appeared in the cancer mortality statistics — are alive today because of medical advances.

Despite this progress, cancer remains a chilling prospect. Cancer actually comprises a large group of diseases, all of which are characterized by uncontrolled growth and spread of abnormal cells. Unchecked proliferation of cancerous cells causes the death of the infested organism.

One out of every five deaths in the U.S. is a cancer victim. In 1984, 450,000 Americans died of this disease, which is second only to heart disease among the leading killers of Americans. Each day, 1,230 people die of cancer; this represents about one death every seventy seconds.

In a recent study of 3,214 deaths among mental institution patients in Texas, researchers discovered that only 4 percent died from cancer. The average rate for the general population in the U.S. is 18 percent.

Cancer can strike anyone at any age. Although more prevalent among the elderly, cancer kills more children ages three to fourteen than any other disease. In the period 1970-1979, cancer was responsible for an estimated 3.5 million deaths in the U.S. and more than 6.5 million new cancer cases were reported during this period. Approximately 30 percent of the current U.S. population — 67 million people — will eventually contract cancer. There are more than 5 million people alive today who have a history of cancer, 3 million of whom are considered "cured," having survived five years or longer.

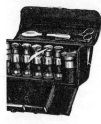

When average U.S. life expectancy is taken into consideration —excluding cancer-diagnosed patients who die of other causes, e.g., heart disease, auto accidents, etc. — then 48 percent of the cancer patients will be alive five years after diagnosis. This is called the "relative" survival rate and it is the most commonly used standard of measuring progress against this disease.

Death is known to occur from over-use of such non-prescription medication as aspirin, analgesics, laxatives, and antihistamines.

Unfortunately, the cancer rate continues to rise. In 1930, the national cancer death rate was 143 (the number of cancer deaths per 100,000 population). In 1940 the rate was 152; in 1950, 158. By 1980, the rate had increased to 169. The major factor responsible for this increase is lung cancer.

While all other types of cancers are leveling off or declining, the death rate for lung cancer has increased tenfold since 1930. In 1984, 139,000 Americans contracted lung cancer and the disease killed 121,000 Americans that year. Chances of surviving this disease are among the bleakest of the cancers: only 9 percent of diagnosed patients survive five or more years.

Still, lung cancer is considered one of the few preventable types of cancer. Medical authorities concur that smoking is the primary cause of lung cancer, accounting for 75 percent of the deaths. More than 90,000 needless deaths will occur in 1984 due to smoking. Lung cancer then, is not invincible.

One of the deadliest diseases in the world is Japanese River Fever, with a mortality rate of more than 50 percent. It is found only near rivers in certain areas of Japan, China, Korea, Formosa, Burma, and India.

———WHERE IN THE U.S. CANCER STRIKES MOST AND LEAST

As the second leading cause of death in the U.S., the cancer death rate for 1980 was 183.9 nationally. The Rocky Mountain region had the lowest rate with 136.4, while the Middle Atlantic region had the highest, 214.7.

Overall, Alaska is the state with the lowest death rate from cancer — for 1980, a rate of 70.2. Utah was second with a rate of 93.6.

Washington, D.C., has the dubious distinction of being number one on the cancer death rate list, with a 1980 rate of 251.6. The state of Florida came in second highest with a rate of 243.0, and third place Pennsylvania had a rate of 220.1.

When tea first became available in Europe in the sixteenth century, some physicians warned that it would bring an early death to those who drank it, especially if they were older than forty.

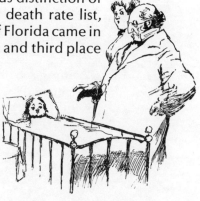

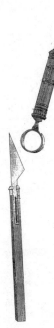

CANCER SURVIVAL INCREASING

Today, more than half of those struck by cancer can expect to survive for more than five years. This represents a dramatic increase in cancer survival rates from the previous two decades. Some credit for this can be given to the federal government's $9.6 billion cancer program which, over the past ten years, increased the number of cancer specialists in the U.S. tenfold.

U.S. SURVIVAL RATES (5 YEARS OR MORE)

Type Of Cancer	Percent Surviving Diagnosed In	
	1960-63	1973-80
Lining of Uterus	73	87
Testis	63	82
Melanoma of skin	60	79
Breast	63	73
Bladder	53	72
Hodgkin's disease	40	70
Uterine cervix	58	67
Prostate	50	67
Colon	43	50
Kidney	37	50
Rectum	38	48
Non-Hodgkin's lymphoma	31	46
Ovary	32	37
Leukemia	14	32
Brain	18	22
Stomach	11	15
Lung	8	12
Among Children		
Hodgkin's disease	52	84
Wilm's tumor	57	75
Acute lymphatic leukemia	4	58
Brain/central nervous system	35	53
Neuroblastoma	25	47
Bone	20	46

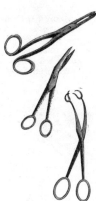

WORLDWIDE CANCER DEATH RATES

DEADLIEST COUNTRIES	DEATH RATE (per 100,000)
Scotland	266.7
West Germany	263.9
Denmark	259.0

LEAST DEADLY COUNTRIES	
Honduras	17.6
Jordan	10.8
Syria	8.2

(The U.S. ranks thirteenth worldwide: 183.9 fatalities per 100,000 population.)

INFANT/MATERNAL MORTALITY

"Death is the price paid by life for an enhancement of the complexity of a live organism's structure."
— Arnold Toynbee

Among the most significant achievements of modern medical science has been the dramatic reduction of infant mortalities and maternal mortalities associated with pregnancy and childbirth.

Reliable records of this data were first assembled in 1915 in the U.S. and during the next five years, 100 out of 1,000 infants did not survive the first year of life. During the same period, between sixty and ninety-two mothers died in childbirth for every 1,000 live births recorded.

During the food shortages of World War II in Germany, the infant mortality rate in Berlin escalated to 359 fatalities per thousand, several times higher than that of underdeveloped countries today.

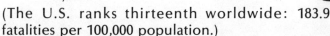

This compares to 1980 statistics for the U.S. of 12.6 infant deaths per 1,000 live births, and 9.2 maternal deaths per 1,000 live births. In 1980, 3,612,000 live births occurred in the U.S., of which 45,511 infants died during the first year. With the infant mortality rate of 1915, 361,000 infants would not have survived their first year of life.

Approximately 33,230 women died in childbirth in 1980, compared to 333,000 who might have died had the death rate been the same as in 1915. These two factors have made a significant impact on vital statistics in general, and have helped widen the gap in the longevity differential between men and women.

Sudden infant death syndrome (crib death) kills one baby in 750.

THE RAVAGES OF INFECTIOUS DISEASES

"Any one not coming to be a dead one before coming to be an old one comes to be an old one and comes then to be a dead one as any old one comes to be a dead one."
— Gertrude Stein

The spread of infectious diseases — often accompanied by devastating death tolls — has continued unabated for centuries. Not until Pasteur identified the microorganisms that cause such diseases, and the conditions under which these parasites flourished and were transmitted, was man able to bring infectious disease somewhat under control. Finally, the development of antibiotics and vaccines turned the statistics around. In 1900, for example, the three major communicable diseases in

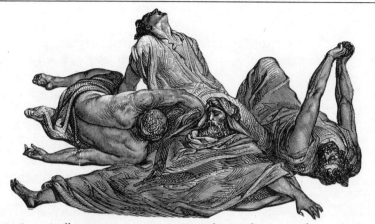

the U.S. — influenza/pneumonia, tuberculosis, and gastritis — held sway as the three leading causes of death. By 1960, however, these three accounted for less than five percent of all deaths in the U.S.

While bacterial parasites can be identified as the specific agents that cause most of these infections, the epidemic proportions of these silent and sudden killers can be attributed to a combination of evolutionary and historical circumstances.

A widely accepted theory places mankind's evolution in tropical rain forests where microorganisms thrived concurrently. Early man therefore evolved with immunity to a wide variety of such parasites. When humans began to migrate to other parts of the world, they wandered into the drier, colder regions — locales where microorganisms were less prolific and not nearly as abundant as in the tropics. Outside of the original habitat, people gradually lost their immunity from these infectious agents. But, as long as man remained a nomadic hunter, he was probably healthy and relatively unsusceptible to microparasitic disease.

However, the creation of civilization — large groups of people settling in particular areas, beginning agricultural practices, and domesticating animals — provided an environment in which

Typhoid Mary died in 1938 while under detention on North Brother Island on the East River in New York City. Seven separate typhoid epidemics were linked to her. Estimates of deaths resulting from her spread of the disease ranged from a few hundred to more than 1,000.

Franz Schubert, classical composer, died in 1828 from tyhphoid fever.

Lou Gehrig, baseball player, died in 1941 of amyotrophic lateral sclerosis, a rare disease which subsequently came to be known as "Lou Gehrig's Disease."

According to a report from a doctor in Great Britain, a ten-year-old girl who had a habit of pulling out her hair and eating it, died in 1982 from peritonitis. An autopsy revealed that her stomach was full of hair.

microorganisms could flourish. By now no longer immune to diseases, these early peoples lived among their animals, their foodstuffs, their garbage, and their sewage — all concentrated in one location. Introduction of bacterial diseases into such densely packed areas could create dire results, in many cases, killing half the population or more. This devastation could continue for a few generations until an immunity to the disease was established among the general population.

Most, if not all, infectious diseases were initially transmitted to human populations by animals. With the creation of civilization came the domestication of herd and pack animals, and microorganisms thrived in these animals. Man came in constant contact with domesticated breeds, ate them, touched them, slept with them, and wore them. It is not surprising then that most of our infectious diseases have a recognizable counterpart in one or another of the diseases of domesticated animals.

It is believed that measles are probably related to *Rinderpest*, or *canine distemper*, and smallpox is surely related to *cowpox*. Flu is suffered by both humans and pigs. Almost everyone is aware of the source of rabies. Rodents have long been verified as the source of bubonic plague. In fact, small outbreaks of bubonic plague, generally transmitted by the fleas on small mammals and bats, still occur in the American West.

Indeed, humans share many types of diseases with a variety of domestic animals. Below, a listing of domestic animals and the number of diseases they have in common with humans:

POULTRY	26	PIGS	42
RATS & MICE	32	SHEEP & GOATS	46
HORSES	35	DOGS	65

In October, 1977, the World Health Organization announced that smallpox had been eradicated from the earth. Only ten years earlier more than 2 million people died from this disease in a single year.

(Persistent rumors that syphilis came from sexual contact with sheep and gonorrhea originated from sexual contact with llamas are still being studied.)

But another factor was necessary to introduce the infectious agent responsible for epidemics into an isolated, stationary civilized population — a population that lacked immunity. For a microorganism to be transported from one geographical location to another required the movement of a large group of people from one location, where the bacteria was established and the local population immune, to another location, where the population was not immune. The most common such event was a military invasion.

The Black Plague (bubonic plague epidemic) that raged worldwide from 1348 to 1361 was transported by Genghis Khan and his Mongol hordes. They invaded Europe from the western steppes of Mongolia, decimating perhaps half the world's population or more within thirteen years.

Likewise, when the Europeans invaded the Americas, they brought with them diseases to which they were immune, but with which the Mexican Indians had no experience. In less than fifty years, infectious diseases — smallpox, measles, and typhus — transmitted by these conquering heroes reduced the native population from 30 million to 3 million. From 1556 to 1560, an influenza outbreak annihilated another 20 percent of the native inhabitants, and by 1620, the indigenous population was reduced to 1.6 million. When malaria came to the New World in 1648, it obliterated almost all of

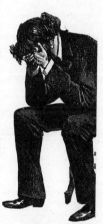

In less than thirteen years, from 1348 to 1361, the bubonic plague may have cut the population of the world in half.

the remaining Indian population, leaving less than half-a-million. Within 150 years, the infec-tious diseases introduced by military invasions destroyed more than 98 percent of the native American population.

The only means of transporting these diseases that rivaled military invasions was religious pilgrim-ages. As with the invasions, these journeys also created a set of circumstances necessary for epidemics: large numbers of people moving from one location to another — accompanied by their invisible local parasites that would eagerly attach themselves to the new, unprotected hosts of a different geographical region.

While in recent years fatalities caused by epidemics have been greatly reduced through international efforts in immunization, antibiotics, and improved sanitation, epidemics of influenza (flu) have swept across the world several times in the past three decades.

These worldwide flu epidemics, caused by a viral agent which is unresponsive to antibiotics, spread rapidly because of the highly mobile nature of the modern global community. Within a three-year period, the "Asian flu," as it was called, was responsible for as many as 86,000 deaths between 1957 and 1960, with 40,000 deaths being attributed to the first wave of this epidemic (September through December, 1957). An additional 20,000 fatalities occurred between January and March 1958, and the third wave, January through March of 1960, brought an additional 27,000 deaths. In many cases, death certificates did not credit influenza as the direct cause of death, but flu was regarded as the underlying cause in numerous cases of death attributed to pneumonia and renal, cardiovascular fatalities.

Al Capone died died from an untreated, advanced case of syphilis in 1947. Other famous deaths from this social disease were Heinrich Heine, the German poet, who expired in 1856, and Guy de Maupassant, writer, who died in 1893. De Maupassant had written earlier, "I am in my death agony. I have a softening of the brain brought on by bathing my nostrils with salt water. The salt has fermented in my brain, and every night my brains are dripping away through my nose and mouth in a sticky paste."

EPIDEMICS OF OLD

In 1947, an epidemic of trichinosis killed thirty-three Eskimos. This parasite is transmitted to humans from contaminated meat, usually raw or under-cooked. The Eskimos had been eating raw polar bear meat.

Our most familiar references to plagues, pestilence, and epidemic disease come from the Bible. Although these texts were written long after the actual events, they represent oral traditions with probable historical bases. In the Book of Exodus, Moses brought down upon Egypt various plagues, wreaking death and destruction. Exodus also describes an epidemic visited upon the Philistines for their violation of the Ark.

Later, if we can believe the chronicler, David's sin was punished by a plague that took 70,000 of the 1,300,000 able-bodied men of Israel. Reference is also made to that fatal visitation which "slew in the camp of the Assyrians 185,000 overnight," causing the Assyrians to retreat from Judea without capturing Jerusalem.

The Bible is not the only source of information about ancient plagues and pestilence. Thucydides describes an epidemic that occurred in 430-429 B.C., "The infection first began, it is said, in the parts of Ethiopia above Egypt and thence descended into Egypt and Libya and into most of the King's country, Persia. Suddenly falling upon Athens, it first attacked the population of Piraeus ... and afterwards appeared in the upper city where the deaths became much more frequent."

The Romans were subject to numerous epidemics. Livy recorded eleven cases in Republican times, the earliest of which he dated at 387 B.C. Another struck in 65 A.D., but the most severe epidemic of Roman times came in 165 A.D. This epidemic was brought back to Rome from troops campaigning in Mesopotamia. A number of subsequent epidemics

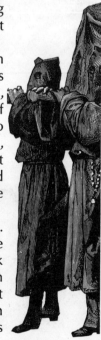

involving the first introduction of smallpox and measles into the Mediterranean had an important effect on the cultural and political deterioration of the Roman Empire.

Finally, in 542 A.D., the "Plague of Justinian" struck the Roman Empire, continuing its rage until 750. It is regarded as the first establishment of bubonic plague in the Mediterranean. At the peak of its first visitation, it swept through Constantinople, lasted four months, and killed 10,000 every day. Some historians regard this epidemic as the final straw in the decline of the Roman Empire: its weakened state made it indefensible against the Moslem invaders. The subsequent shift of important European historical centers and capitals northward, away from tropical climates, is also considered a result of the Plague of Justinian.

Thus, some maintain that disease — more than military might, despotic personalities, religious proselytization, weapons technology, cultural evolution, or any other factor — had the greatest influence on the evolution of civilization, the creation and destruction of empires, and the shaping of the modern world.

Daniel D. Tompkins, sixth Vice President of the U.S., died in 1825, after writing that he suffered from, "toilsome days, sleepless nights, anxious cares, domestic bereavements, impaired constitution, debilitated body, unjust abuse and censure, and accumulated pecuniary embarrassments."

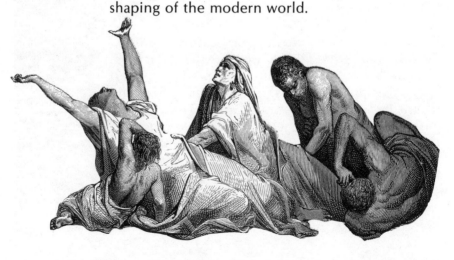

EPIDEMICS
AND PLAGUES

"Do not go gentle into that good night.
Rage, rage against the dying of the light."
— Dylan Thomas

During World War I, influenza killed more soldiers than all the weapons combined.

Until after the turn of this century, communicable diseases constituted the primary cause of death worldwide. Historically, epidemics of contagious diseases, including the plague, have caused more deaths in shorter amount of time, than all other causes of death combined. Nothing in modern times can begin to compare with epidemic death tolls of the past.

As many as 30,000 people may die every year from adverse reactions to antibiotics.

Century	Type	Place	Fatalities
500	Bubonic plague	Europe, Asia	100 million
1000-1100	(Unknown)	Europe	300,000
1300-1400	Bubonic plague	World	27 million
1400-1500	Bubonic plague	Paris	
	Sweating sickness	England	100,000
1500-1600	Sweating sickness	England	
	Smallpox	Mexico	
	Measles	Mexico	
	(Unknown)	Mexico	10 million
1600-1700	Bubonic plague	London, Europe	
	Typhus	Europe	500,000
1700-1800	Bubonic plague	Europe, Russia	600,000
1800-1900	Bubonic plague	China, India	
	Yellow fever	Haiti	
	Measles, malaria	South Pacific islands	
	Cholera	Europe, Russia	
	Typhus	Canada	300,000
1900-1985	Bubonic plague	India, China	
	Malaria	India	
	Cholera	Russia, Egypt	
	Typhus	Russia, Poland	
	Dysentery	Poland	
	Influenza	Worldwide	37 million

DRUGS AND LIFE EXPECTANCY

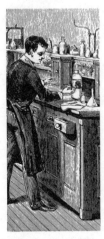

Penicillin
causes about
300 deaths
every year in
the U.S.

"The fundamental precept of the fight for longevity is avoidance of satiation. One must not lose desires. They are mighty stimulants to creativeness, to love, and to long life."
— St. Thomas Aquinas

Not only do the Japanese live longer than most other people, they also spend more on drugs. The longer life expectancy of the Japanese (76 years) is matched only by those living in Iceland and Hong Kong. Drug expenditures in Japan equal $94 per capita per year.

The table below demonstrates how this correlation — between expenses for drugs and medical care and longevity — can be found in most countries. The figures below, representing the 1981 world drug market, were compiled by the London-based IMS group.

	Drug Expenditure per Capita (In U.S. Dollars)	Life Expectancy At Birth
Japan	94.18	76
West Germany	88.71	72
Switzerland	78.73	73
France	77.80	73
U.S.A.	70.88	73
Belgium	67.67	71
Sweden	61.33	75
Argentina	58.67	69
Great Britain	45.88	72
Australia	39.43	73
Spain	39.15	72
Brazil	10.57	64
India	1.30	52

THE GOOD OLD DAYS

Before the discovery and widespread adoption of anesthetics and sanitation in the operating room, there was seldom more than a fifty-fifty chance of surviving most operations. A statistical report from the mid-1800s listed these fatality rates from amputations:

Forearm	13 percent
Arm	52
Leg	50
Thigh	85

Joseph Lister, founder of modern antiseptic surgery, was responsible more than any other for cleaning up the deadly statistics of the surgeons. A comparison made of before-and-after fatality rates in one hospital clearly shows what progress can do.

AMPUTATION	FATALITY RATE	
	Old System	Lister System
Arm	10 percent	0 percent
Leg	33	2
Thigh	41	7
Shoulder	52	11
General	30	4

In Babylonia, circa 3,000 B.C., physicians who were responsible for the death of their patients had their hands cut off, unless the patient was a slave, in which case the doctor was required to replace him with one of his own slaves.

The atomic bomb explosion at Hiroshima killed or injured 90 percent of the city's doctors; 86 percent of its dentists; 80 percent of its pharmacists; and 93 percent of its nurses.

DEAD AND BURIED

During the nineteenth century, many people shared a deep fear of being buried while unconscious and presumed dead. Many devices and methods were developed to test corpses for the permanence of the death state, one of the most practical being a large pair of tongs which were

A famous surgeon from nineteenth century England named Liston set a record by amputating the leg of a patient in less than two-and-a-half minutes. Unfortunately, the spectacle was too much for another doctor who was observing; he died from a stroke. The patient also died later from gangrene — as did a surgical assistant whose fingers were mistakenly amputated in the same operation.

used to pinch the nipples of male and female bodies and possibly elicit a response. During the relocation of some cemeteries, it was discovered that numerous people had been buried alive, and suffocated while trying to escape from their coffins. Corpses found in such tortured conditions may have been responsible for the vampire myths in earlier centuries.

___DOCTOR ERRORS

"Death can take all ills away;
But here we are, and here would stay.
'Better to suffer than to die'
Is Everyman's philosophy."
— Jean de la Fontaine

Health care technology may have become more effective, but doctors can still make mistakes. A recent study was conducted at two Boston hospitals to compare the results of postmortem examinations from 1960, 1970, and 1980. The object was to determine how accurate patient diagnosis was. In each year studied, it was discovered that about 10 percent of the patients had been mis-diagnosed in such a manner as to have affected the possibility of survival. Another 12 percent of the cases each year also had included diagnostic errors, but not to an extent that would have affected the patients' chances of surviving.

The researchers responsible for this study believe that advanced diagnostic methods and treatments have improved over the years, but in some cases left room for infections and diseases to attack without being noticed while major symptoms were being dealt with. Autopsies are the best tool for determining missed diagnoses, but they have become more expensive, time consuming, and they increase the risk of malpractice lawsuits. The autopsy rate is currently about 15 percent.

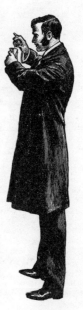

CURED TO DEATH

Statistics from modern hospitals suggest a strange possibility, that often a treatment can be more fatal than an illness. In hospitals associated with teaching programs, there is often a higher mortality rate than in non-teaching hospitals. In one study, there was a fatality rate for neo-natal cases that was 30 percent higher in teaching hospitals than in others, and a rate for maternal deaths that was 200 percent higher (26.3 deaths per 100,000 compared to 52.1 deaths per 100,000).

These differences might be attributed to error, carelessness, or even the tendency for experimentation and unnecessary procedures that are performed when medical students are involved, as opposed to conserving treatment to only what is necessary in non-teaching hospitals. If so, the more medical treatment you receive from student doctors, the more likely you might expire.

In Great Britain, where similar statistics have been found to be true, results show that it is actually safer for a mother to give birth at home than in a hospital, even though the medical community there discourages this practice.

A bronchial inhaler in widespread use in England in the 1960s was responsible for an epidemic of fatalities in children who had the inhalers prescribed for treatment of asthma.

_____NOISE DEATHS

"Death has got something to be said for it:
There's no need to get out of bed for it;
Wherever you may be,
They bring it to you, free."
— Kingsley Amis

In 1983 at a church in a small town in Ohio, a minister delivered his own eulogy. After battling cancer for two years, the reverend recorded the sermon on videotape, anticipating his impending death.

At least one scientific study has been done to indicate a direct link between noise and cardiovascular disease. In the early 1980s, two communities in the vicinity of the Los Angeles airport were studied. Both communities were similar in characteristics for socio-economic levels, population, and racial makeup. However, while one region had a minimum level of outdoor jet noise of 90 decibels (dB) — industrial workers exposed to this level of noise are required to wear protective hearing devices — and occasional maximum levels as high as 115 dB, the other area averaged only 50 dB.

In the community with high levels of noise, the mortality rate from heart attacks was 18 percent higher than in the quieter community for residents 75 years of age and older. In addition, there were twice as many suicides in the 45 to 54-year-old age group in the former area (thirty compared to fifteen). Violent deaths, which include murder and automobile accidents as well as suicide, were 60 percent higher in the noisier area for the 75-year-old and older crowd.

The noisy area under study was exposed to more than 650 incoming flights every day, with flights as frequent as every two-and-a-half minutes during peak periods. Because the decibel scale is logarithmic in character, every increase in decibel level results in an increase of sound pressure much greater than the decibel increase. The difference between the 50 dB level in the quieter neighborhood and the 90 dB in the noisy one therefore resulted in an increase in sound pressure of more than 10,000 times.

Researchers theorize that since earlier studies have shown that blood pressure can be affected by loud noises, this airport noise study indicates that sustained exposure to high levels of noise can increase the risk of heart attacks, strokes, and related cardiovascular problems, plus the death rate associated with these health problems.

Charlie Parker, jazz saxophonist, died from pneumonia in 1955 at the age of thirty-three, but the coroner estimated the age of the body at fifty to sixty years old.

WHERE PEOPLE DIE

More than half of all deaths occur in hospitals. When nursing homes and similar health institutions are included, about 75 percent of all deaths are accounted for. If the location of all deaths in the U.S. is taken into account, then an appropriate definition of hospital might be: a place where people go to die.

Heart attacks are the least discriminating health problems in choosing their spot. Only 50 percent of heart failures occur inside formal health care facilities. Infant diseases are most localized, with about 95 percent occurring in hospitals and related institutions.

During Napolean's Penninsula Campaign, the French lost 400,000 troops to disease, and only 60,000 in battle.

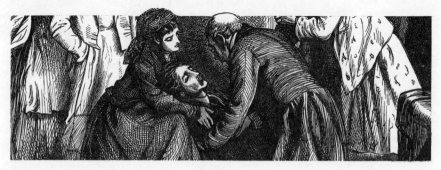

"Death be not proud, though some have called thee
Mighty and dreadful, for thou art not so,
For, those, whom thou think'st, thou dost overthrow,
Die not, poor death, nor yet canst thou kill me . . .
. . . death, thou shalt die."
— John Donne

Chapter Three

SLIPPERY WHEN WET
Death from Accidents

Accidents are the fourth leading cause of death nationwide and among all age groups — accounting for about 100,000 fatalities annually. About half of these deaths can be attributed to motor vehicle accidents; about one-third occur in the home.

Heart disease, cancer, and stroke all take more lives annually among all age groups, but accidents are the leading cause of death among all persons age one to thirty-eight. Every hour of every day of the year, eleven people die of accidental death and another 1,070 suffer disabling injuries.

In the U.S., accidental deaths reached a peak in 1969 with 116,385 fatalities. Between 1969 and 1974, the vehicular death toll hovered at about 55,000 annually. But since the enactment of the nationwide 55 mile-per-hour speed limit in late 1973, the traffic death toll has been dramatically reduced in subsequent years; a corresponding decrease in the overall accidental death rate has also taken place. Since 1969, accident fatalities have continued to decrease.

ACCIDENT FACTS

"I am one of those unfortunates to whom
death is less hideous than explanations."
— D. B. Wyndham Lewis

Worst Places to Be — Highest fatalities per 100,000
population:

STATES

1. Alaska   103.2
2. Wyoming   88.8
3. Montana   75.3
4. Mississippi   71.4
5. Nevada   69.8

CITIES

1. New London, Connecticut   127.9
2. Saginaw, Michigan   114.8
3. Oklahoma City, Oklahoma   90.2
4. Tulsa, Oklahoma   76.9
5. Seattle, Washington   63.0

Safest Places to Be — Lowest fatalities:

STATES

1. New Jersey   23.9
2. Delaware   26.3
3. New York   27.3
4. Pennsylvania   30.1
5. Maryland   31.7

CITIES

1. Allentown, Pennsylvania   9.4
2. New Haven, Connecticut   12.6
3. New York, New York   16.8
4. Independence, Missouri   17.9
5. Rockford, Illinois   18.6

New Jersey has the lowest death rate from accidents of all the states of the union — 23.9 accident fatalities per 100,000 population. Alaska has the highest rate — 103.2 accident fatalities per 100,000.

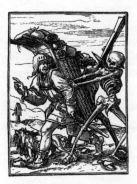

A mass panic at a soccer game in Buenos Aires, Argentina, in 1968, left seventy-one people dead.

In 1983, a one-year-old child in Colorado was killed in an accident with a toilet. The child had been playing next to the toilet; the lid fell, knocking him unconscious and trapping his head. Death was due to asphyxiation.

Most Fatal Month   **July**
Least Fatal Month   **February**
Most Fatal Sex   **Male**
Most Fatal Age   **Older than 75 years**
Least Fatal Age   **5-14 years**

Most Deadly Accidents:

1. **Automobile**
2. **Falls**
3. **Drowning**

Worst month for poison   **January**
Worst month for falls   **January**
Worst month for drowning   **July**
Worst month for choking   **January**
Worst month for gassing   **January**

Aspirin had killed more than one hundred children under the age of five every year in the U.S. until tamper-proof caps made this common medicine harder to get to. The average is now fewer than fifty deaths per year.

Men have more accidents than women — of the total, these are the percentages claimed by males:

Falls	52 percent
Drowning	84 percent
Fires/burns	61 percent
Choking	58 percent
Firearms	87 percent
Poisons	59 percent
Gas	73 percent

☐ Since 1912, the death rate from accidents has dropped by about half.
☐ On the average, about eleven people die every hour from accidents.
☐ In 1928, 32 percent of all accidental deaths occurred in the home.
☐ In 1981, 21 percent were in the home.
☐ In 1928, 20 percent of all accidental deaths occurred at work.
☐ In 1981, 12 percent were at work.

The first railroad bridge fatality in the U.S. was on March 4, 1840, at High Rock Bridge in New York.

Five deadliest nations for accidents:
1. Luxembourg   69.6 fatal accidents per
                                100,000 people
2. Hungary   67.1
3. Austria   62.7
4. Venezuela   61.6
5. Northern Ireland   56.2

Five least deadly nations:
1. Singapore   15.4 fatal accidents per
                                100,000 people
2. Dominican Republic   18.4
3. Hong Kong   24.5
4. Japan   25.0
5. Nicaragua   29.8

No one in the U.S. has been electrocuted while talking on the phone in a bathtub or shower. However, conditions could exist that would produce lethal voltage from a telephone, and the phone company does not recommend this combination of activities.

Since 1912, the death rate from accidents at work has dropped more than 75 percent in the U.S.
Most fatal industry: **Mining** (55 deaths per 100,000 workers)
Least fatal industry: **Wholesale and retail trade** (5 deaths per 100,000 workers)

ANNUAL FATALITIES FROM ACCIDENTS

	Total Fatalities	Death Rate (per 100,000)
1970	114,638	56.2
1975	103,030	48.4
1980	105,700	46.7

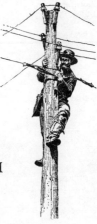

LEADING CAUSES OF ACCIDENTAL DEATH

	1975	1980
All Accidental Deaths	103,030	105,000
Motor Vehicle	45,853	52,600
Falls	14,896	13,400
Fires and Flames	6,071	5,500
Drowning	6,640	7,000
Poisoning	6,271	4,300
Other Transportation	3,985	4,511

WHERE ACCIDENTS HAPPEN

Bedrooms are the scene for 40 percent of all accidents in the home; another 12 percent happen in the kitchens, 10 percent in living rooms, 4 percent on staircases, 3 percent in bathrooms, 3 percent in dining rooms, and 1 percent in basements.

Another means of evaluating accidental death statistics is to find out where the fatalities occur — at home, in the workplace, or in public. Excluding motor vehicle fatalities, year after year, more accidental deaths have occurred in the home than at work or in public — probably because most people spend more time at home than anywhere else. All three locations of accidental deaths have shown a steady decline since the beginning of the century. Here is a breakdown for 1980:

Auto	Work	Home	Public	Total
52,600	13,000	23,000	21,700	105,700

In London in 1964 a crane lifting a building section that weighed more than seven tons collapsed. The section fell on a bus and killed seven passengers.

WORLD ACCIDENT FATALITIES

More than 1,000 people die every year from falling objects.

	Fatalities	Rate (per 100,000)
Hong Kong	1,240	24.5
Japan	29,217	25.0
Nicaragua	718	29.8
Britain	14,854	30.2
Israel	1,196	32.4
Sweden	3,610	43.5
West Germany	28,374	46.2
United States	99,000	43.2
Scotland	2,545	49.3
Poland	19,241	54.3
Hungary	7,176	67.1
Luxembourg	253	69.6

FIRE FATALITIES

"The weariest and most loathed worldly life
That age, ache, penury, and imprisonment
Can lay on nature, is a paradise
To what we fear of death."
— Shakespeare

Combustible materials have a long history of turning men into ashes. Even excluding spectacular conflagrations that kill many people, the current leader in the U.S. among accident killers is fire. Specifically, the burning of upholstery and mattresses from smokers causes more fatalities every year than any other type of mishap. This grim statistic is not shared by most countries of the world, because not every country mimics the U.S. tobacco industry's habit of adding chemicals to cigarettes to keep them lit. For this characteristic and their destructive influence on human health, they can aptly be nicknamed, "coffin nails."

Nine women, patients at a mental institution in Cleveland, Ohio, died in 1933 in a fire that consumed the building where they were housed. Although the fire was discovered in time and the patients led to safety, they apparently found the night air too cold and their night clothes too thin so they ran back inside to get warm by the fire.

More than 16,000 people die from falls every year in the U.S.

FIRE STATS

Deadliest place for fires: **homes**
Deadliest state (death rate per population): **Alaska**
Least deadly state: **Hawaii**
Most frequent source of fatal fires: **smoking** — ignition of upholstered furniture most often, closely followed by ignition of mattresses

About 36 percent of all firefighter fatalities occur in non-fire situations.

Deadliest time: **midnight to 4:00 A.M.**
Least deadly time: **4:00 P.M. to 8:00 P.M.**
Deadliest ages: **more than sixty and less than ten years of age**
Least deadly ages: **thirty-to-forty years of age**
Most frequent cause of death from fires: **burns and smoke inhalation**
Most frequent victim: **non-white males**
Least frequent victims: **white females**
Major cause of death of fire fighters: **heart attack** (50 percent of all fatalities)
Average loss of life from fire in the U.S. per year: **7,000**
Average firefighter deaths in the U.S. per year: **100**
Most dangerous country for fires (death rate per population): **Canada** (U.S. is second)
Safest country: **The Netherlands**

On April 18, 1984, an elephant named Ellie was electrocuted while in the process of erecting a circus tent. The tent pole she was lifting contacted a power line, which supplied the fatal jolt. As Ellie collapsed, she crushed her trainer to death.

A general rule of thumb for fatalities from burns: the percent of mortality is about the same as the percent of body area that has been burned. That is, when sixty percent of the body is burned, death will result about sixty percent of the time. However, the age of the victim is an important factor in chances of survival. Another general rule of thumb: if the percent of body area burned plus the age of the patient is greater than 100, the victim will probably die.

In 1962, a window-washing scaffold fell nineteen stories from the side of the Equitable Building in New York City. Four men who were working on the platform were killed.

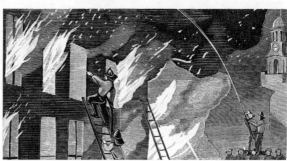

—FIRE FATALITIES IN THE U.S.

Among the notable structure fires in U.S. history which have taken multiple lives are these:

		Fatalities
Iroquois Theater, Chicago, Illinois	December 30, 1903	602
Coconut Grove Night Club, Boston, Mass.	November 28, 1942	492
Ohio State Penitentiary, Columbus, Ohio	April 21, 1930	320
London High School, London, Texas	March 18, 1937	294
Lake View School, Collinwood, Ohio	March 4, 1908	175
Rhodes Opera House, Boyertown, Penn.	January 12, 1903	170
Ringling Brothers Circus, Hartford, Conn.	July 6, 1944	168
Beverly Hills Supper Club, Southgate, Kent.	May 28, 1977	165
Triangle Shirtwaist Co. New York City	March 25, 1911	145

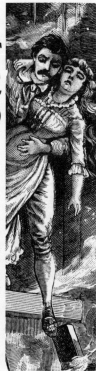

—————WORST FIRES IN THE WORLD

"I do not want to achieve immortality through my work . . . I want to achieve it through not dying."
— Woody Allen

		Fatalities
Moscow, Russia	1570	200,000
Cairo, Egypt	1824	4,000
Santiago, Chile	1863	1,800
Chungking, China	Sep. 2, 1949	1,700
Vienna, Austria	Dec.8, 1881	620
Abadan, Iran	Aug. 20, 1978	400
Niteroi, Brazil	Dec. 17, 1961	323
Brussels, Belgium	May 22, 1967	322
Sao Paulo, Brazil	Feb. 1, 1974	189
St.-Laurent-du-Pont, France	Nov. 1, 1970	146

DEATH ON THE JOB

"No one owns life, but anyone who can pick up a frying pan owns death."
— William Burroughs

In July, 1981, an industrial worker died from radiation poisoning in Oklahoma. According to government records, this is the first death in the U.S. from radiation poisoning since the development of the atom bomb.

Progress in the industrial world has not been achieved without suffering. Loss of life in the construction industries has always been high. Even with modern safety measures and high worker standards, accidents take a significant toll of life.

During the Spanish-American War, the U.S. lost 385 lives in battle. During that same period, in one county of Pennsylvania alone, there were 520 industrial accidents. In recent years, industrial accidents have accounted for an average of 12,000 deaths per year in the U.S. Most of these are in the construction industry; manufacturing is a close second. When occupation-related diseases are included, the annual death rate is estimated to be about 100,000.

The digging of a tunnel in Gauley Bridge, West Virginia, in 1930 resulted in the deaths of more than 475 workers from inhalation of silica dust. Many of them were black, and they were buried in a field, several to a hole.

Agriculture can be deceptive in its danger. Most fatalities in farming occur from equipment accidents; most of these are from moving implements. However, grain dust explosions cause larger losses of life in single accidents — such explosions are as powerful and as lethal as explosions from gases or explosives. Since 1900, more than 550 people have been killed by explosions in grain elevators in the U.S. In Australia, this problem is almost non-existent; stringent practices are followed to prevent the build-up of dangerous amounts of dust in grain facilities.

These are some of the facts about job-related accidents:

Deadliest work day | **Tuesday**
Safest work day | **Friday**
Deadliest work month | **July**
Safest work month | **February**
Deadliest occupation | **Trucking**
Safest occupation | **Retail sales**
Deadliest state | **Texas**
Safest state | **Delaware**
Deadliest aspect of all types of work | **Transportation**

In 1930, thirty people died in Bombay, India, from eating soup made from a poisonous lizard.

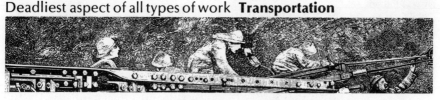

POP GOES THE WEASEL

Dynamite isn't the only thing that blows up people who are in the way; there is a long and gruesome history of other substances that have exploded and taken lives. Whenever an explosion occurs, most deaths are a result of the tremendous pressures generated by the blast and the effects of debris traveling at very high velocities. Lives can also be lost from secondary effects, the most significant one being severe burns.

Some big bangs from history:

A rupture in a tank in a brewery in London in 1814 sent 3,500 barrels of beer flooding through a densely populated area of the city; nine people were killed by this man-made flood.

	Source Of Explosion		Fatalities
Eddystone, Pennsylvania	Munitions	April 10, 1917	133
New London, Texas	Natural gas	March 18, 1937	294
Kenvil, New Jersey	Munitions	September 11, 1940	100
Port Chicago, California	Unknown	July 17, 1944	322
Cleveland, Ohio	Liquid gas	October 20, 1944	135
Texas City, Texas	Ammonium nitrate	April 16, 1947	561
Indianapolis, Indiana	Bottled gas	October 31, 1963	68

MINING DISASTERS IN THE U.S.

There are a few reported cases of fatalities in industrial settings from the use of compressed air to dry hands. In these cases, air was forced into the bloodstream through existing open cuts, and air bubbles in the blood led to death.

Mining disasters attract a lot of attention because of the large number of dead — usually the result of a cave-in or explosion. At the beginning of the twentieth century, there were enough of these events to make mining a very dangerous job, with about 2,000 deaths per year. However, with more modern safety precautions, and more mining being done in the relatively safer surface sites, the real current hazards are health problems associated with working conditions.

According to a report made by a conference of U.S. Mayors in 1936, more Americans have been killed by fireworks celebrating the Fourth of July, than died fighting for the independence of the country in the Revolutionary War. Between the years 1900 and 1930 alone, 4,290 people were killed by fireworks.

There are about 4,000 deaths annually from black lung disease, and about 6,000 deaths are expected over the next two decades from radiation exposure in uranium miners. Silicosis, the most common disease caused by exposure to dust, causes an unknown number of deaths in the mining industry, but its effects are considered to be as lethal as those from black lung. Similarly, asbestosis, a common disease for those often exposed to asbestos, kills miners; however, no estimates are available as to total fatalities.

		Fatalities
Monongah, West Virginia	December 6, 1907	361
Dawson, New Mexico	October 22, 1913	263
Cherry, Illinois	November 13, 1909	259
Jacobs Creek, Pennsylvania	December 19, 1907	239
Scofield, Utah	May 1, 1900	200
Mather, Pennsylvania	May 19, 1928	195
Avondale, Pennsylvania	September 6, 1869	179
Cheswick, Pennsylvania	January 25, 1904	179
West Frankfort, Illinois	December 21, 1951	119

BUILDING FAILURES

"Consistency is contrary to nature, contrary to life. The only completely consistent people are the dead."
— Aldous Huxley

Every year, people are injured and killed while inside buildings — when structural failures cause walls or roofs to collapse. These losses are caused by design errors and material failures, among other things.

Some of the most notable in the U.S. are these:

☐ July 7, 1856: A wharf in Philadelphia, Pennsylvania, collapsed, drowning thirty people.

☐ January 10, 1860: The Pemberton Cotton Mill in Lawrence, Massachusetts, collapsed and burned, killing 117.

☐ April 8, 1873: A crowd of people watching a flood caused a wall to collapse in Rochester, New York, drowning thirty.

☐ May 23, 1877: The Winnebago County Courthouse in Rockford, Illinois, collapsed, killing eleven people.

☐ July 23, 1883: A pier in Baltimore, Maryland, collapsed, drowning seventy people.

☐ August 22, 1891: The Park Place disaster in New York City killed sixty-four.

☐ June 9, 1893: Ford's Theater in Washington, D.C., collapsed, killing twenty-two.

☐ January 28, 1922: The roof of the Knickerbocker Theater in Washington, D.C., collapsed, killing ninety-eight.

☐ July 18, 1981: A walkway at the Hyatt Hotel in Kansas City collapsed, killing 111 people.

In 1919, a huge holding tank containing more than two million gallons of molasses burst open and sent a sea of the sticky substance through a large area of Boston, Massachusetts, hitting buildings and people with a wall of molasses twenty- to thirty-feet high. Twenty-one people died in the Great Boston Molasses Flood.

In thirty fatalities involving spas and hot tubs since 1979, alcohol was a contributing factor in twelve cases, 40 percent of the total.

Sixteen children died in 1983 from accidents related to toys.

_____BREAK STEP!

In 1845, hundreds of people gathered on a suspension bridge over the Bure River in Yarmouth, England, waiting for the arrival of a clown in a small boat, caused the bridge to collapse; seventy-nine people drowned, most of them children.

One of the things that has made modern bridges possible is the all-too-frequent fate of most bridges built before the twentieth century. Bridge builders in days past, generally ignorant of the structural requirements necessary for safety, often resorted to the quickest and least expensive methods of construction.

In the 1800s, using mostly wood and masonry, bridges were required to carry the weight of railroad trains, as well as foot and horse-drawn traffic. Although it was the failure of the expensive and "new-fangled" iron bridges that received the most attention, it wasn't very safe to cross any span in those days, compared to the security we are used to today.

When the Tay Bridge in Scotland collapsed on December 29, 1879, an entire train disappeared into the sea; seventy-five people died.

In one study of bridges in the U.S. in the 1870s, 25 percent self-destructed. An average of forty bridges failed every year in that period; the majority of them were wooden. A report in the *Railway Gazette* from 1895 listed 502 bridge failures associated with trains from 1878 to 1895. Excess weight was not always a factor. One bridge in Massachusetts was known to have collapsed from the weight of a single team of horses.

Dixon, Illinois, the home town of Ronald Reagan, is also known for the collapse of an iron railroad bridge on May 4, 1873; one hundred people died.

A popular misconception has existed throughout history: that marching in unison across a bridge would cause it to collapse. This idea dates back to 1831 when a troop of soldiers marched over a bridge in Broughton, England, apparently causing it to self-destruct. In Angiers, France, in 1850, the worst bridge disaster in history occurred: 200 soldiers died as a bridge collapsed while they were marching across it. Similarly, stories were passed around of smaller, rural bridges that were destroyed when herds of horses or cattle were driven over them. Engineering studies show that most of these catastrophes were caused by inherent structural problems in the bridges.

THERE'S NO SAFETY IN NUMBERS

"Let the dead bury their dead."
— Matthew, VII: 22

On March 4, 1943, 178 people died in an air-raid shelter in London, England — there was a panic from overcrowding and the victims died from suffocation.

When large groups of people assemble, a good time is not necessarily had by all. Hundreds of people have died in the midst of crowds. Although the use of deadly force is most often the cause, just the fact that so many people are in one place at the same time can be fatal to some. Panic can cause people to crowd together so tightly that individuals cannot control what happens to themselves. In many cases, individuals who have fallen have been crushed to death; but more often, the primary cause of death has been a depletion of blood to the brains of those who fainted in the press of bodies.

In London, England, in 1867, the ice on a Regent's Park lake gave way under a crowd of people; more than forty drowned.

Ordinarily, when a person faints, the body slumps and falls to a prone position, which allows blood to circulate freely in the circulatory system. When the body is forcibly held in an upright position, however, the constricted blood vessels in the brain do not get enough blood to maintain necessary functions, and the brain expires.

A Sunday School meeting in Sunderland, England, ended in tragedy on June 15, 1883, when a panic caused a stampede; 200 children died.

		Fatalities
Sunderland, England	June 15, 1883	200
Kyoto, Japan	January 8, 1934	76
London, England	March 4, 1943	178
Lima, Peru	May 25, 1964	218
Buenos Aires, Argentina	June 23, 1968	71
Cairo, Egypt	February 17, 1974	49

*"Death could drop from the dark
As easily as song."*
— Isaac Rosenberg

Chapter Four

ON THE MOVE
Death from Transportation Mishaps

Various methods of transportation have been involved in fatalities since the first man hitched a ride on a horse, but in modern times, we have at least achieved a level of certainty in the possibility of mishaps en route. Standards have gradually risen to guarantee the safety of passengers, starting with government review boards in England in the nineteenth century. Thousands of people drowned at sea before even minimal protection was provided for survival. In the air, where any accident was liable to end in death for most, if not all the passengers on a plane, safety standards were similarly hard won. Railroad travel eclipsed both of these in its adoption of safety procedures only because the first person ever killed by a train was a member of Parliament in England.

In the U.S., the overall number of fatalities from motor vehicle accidents has yet to be equalled by any other country, although stringent safety rules and speed limits have finally brought the domestic fatality rate under control. When compared to the number of vehicles and miles driven in other countries, the U.S. is one of the safest places on earth to drive.

ROAD WARS

"Whenever I prepare for a journey I prepare as though for death. Should I never return, all is in order. This is what life has taught me."
— Katherine Mansfield

As many people die from motor vehicle accidents every year in the U.S. as died fighting for the U.S. in the Vietnam War. This number, about 50,000, is actually an improvement over time since the automobile first became popular, if compared to the total number of miles being driven. In fact, since 1912, the death rate per number of registered vehicles has declined by more than 90 percent.

Currently, there is one motor vehicle death for every 30,400,000 miles driven. Thirty-five percent of all fatal accidents involve a collision between two vehicles. The single largest cause of all fatal accidents is driver error (about 70 percent of the total). Excess speed is the most common fatal mistake. Driving left of center and errors in right-of-way account for about 12 percent each of fatal driving mistakes. Tailgating, improper turns, and passing mistakes account for the remainder.

Motor vehicle accidents — including those that involve fatalities — most often happen close to home. In fact, out of the total number of fatalities, the driver involved lives in the state where the accident occurs more than 80 percent of the time.

Three-fifths of all automobile fatalities occur away from urban areas. This figure reflects the higher rates of speed common away from cities, where denser populations and traffic keep the overall rate of speed down. In addition, more than 60 percent of all fatal accidents occur at night.

Of the total deaths from motor vehicle accidents,

Despite the overall number of fatalities, the U.S. is still the safest country in the world for driving — there are less fatal accidents relative to miles driven and number of people driving than in any other country.

In the USSR, which has only a fraction of the number of automobiles found in the U.S., there are the same number of fatalities every year as here, about 50,000.

more than 60 percent involve passenger cars. Trucks account for about 25 percent of the remainder, motorcycles and motor scooters for 8 percent, and the final 6 percent is split among taxis, buses, farm equipment, and emergency vehicles.

The deadliest drivers: **Males** — Even though both males and females are involved in traffic accidents at about the same rate, two accidents per 100,000 miles driven, male drivers die at twice the rate of females. The difference is generally attributed to the contrast in circumstances involved in the kind of driving done by each sex.

Deadliest day of the week: **Saturday** — This weekend day gets its bum reputation from early morning fatalities related to the closing of bars and other entertainment facilities.

Deadliest hour of the week: **1:00 to 2:00 A.M. Sunday morning** — The Saturday morning syndrome repeated, but condensed into a shorter time frame.

Safest day of the week: **Monday**.

Safest hour of the week: **9:00 to 10:00 A.M. Sunday morning**.

Deadliest month: **August**.

Safest month: **February**.

The deadliest places to drive (highest traffic fatalities in the U.S.):

1. Atlanta, Georgia
2. Nashville, Tennessee
3. Houston, Texas
4. Phoenix, Arizona
5. Dallas, Texas

Accidents in rural areas cause more than twice the fatalities of accidents in urban areas.

The first death from a motor-vehicle accident in the U.S. was on September 13, 1899, when Henry Bliss, age sixty-eight, was hit by an automobile near the corner of 74th Street and Central Park West in New York City.

Two percent of the people killed in accidents between automobiles and trucks are riding in the trucks.

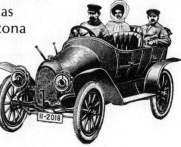

The safest places to drive (lowest traffic fatalities in the U.S.):
1. Boston, Massachusetts
2. Buffalo, New York
3. Washington, D.C.
4. Indianapolis, Indiana
5. Milwaukee, Wisconsin

The deadliest states (highest traffic fatalities in the U.S.):
1. New Mexico
2. Nevada
3. Wyoming
4. Arizona
5. Idaho

The most fatalities from a single automobile crash in the U.S. is eleven, from a wreck near Whitesburg, Kentucky on July 31, 1954.

The deadliest countries (highest traffic fatalities in the world):
1. Portugal
2. Venezuela
3. Canada
4. Australia
5. Belgium
6. West Germany
7. France
8. United States

A streetcar that went out of control in Tacoma, Wasington, on July 4, 1900, killed forty-one people.

The deadliest turnpike (highest traffic fatalities in the U.S.): West Virginia Turnpike.

The safest turnpikes (lowest traffic fatalities in the U.S.):
1. Audubon Parkway, Kentucky
2. Purchase Parkway, Kentucky
3. Dallas North Tollway, Texas
4. Maine Turnpike
5. Florida Turnpike
6. Hutchinson River Parkway, New York

RULES OF THUMB FOR MOTOR VEHICLE FATALITIES

"When life is woe,
And hope is dumb,
The World says, 'Go!'
The Grave says, 'Come!'"
— Arthur Guiterman

If every road in the U.S. had the same rate of motor-vehicle accident fatalities as the Interstate Highway System, there would be 5,000 fewer deaths per year.

Three times more men than women are fatalities in automobile accidents.

The first motorcycle fatality was George Morgan, who fell off his new motor tricycle on February 11, 1899, in Exeter, England.

Traffic fatalities rise when:

□ The economy is prospering. (Even when gasoline prices are high, prosperity induces people to spend money, increasing vehicular travel, producing a corresponding increase in traffic deaths.

□ Drivers switch to smaller cars. (Accidents are more likely to result in fatalities when the vehicles involved are smaller than mid-sized. Less car means less protection.)

□ Vacation time begins. (Every holiday, festival, three-day weekend, and summer break puts more vehicles onto the road, many of them in a hurry to get somewhere for a celebration. Predictably, fatalities are greatest during these periods.)

Traffic fatalities fall when:

□ Gasoline is hard to get. (During the Mideast oil embargo, traffic fatalities fell by more than 18 percent.)

□ Public pressure backs legislation against drunk drivers. (More than 50 percent of all traffic fatalities involve alcohol.)

□ The number of teenage drivers is reduced. (The highest fatality rate for all age groups involved in traffic accidents is teenagers.)

☐ The economy is in a recession. (Hard times place pressure on personal budgets, and one of the first things to suffer is gasoline purchases, especially for vacation and recreation travel.)

☐ The speed limit is lowered. (Speed is the single largest factor in vehicular deaths. When the 55 mile-per-hour speed limit went into effect, fatality rates dropped nationwide.)

In 1966, eleven Belgium students studying traffic safety were killed when a truck ran off the road and smashed into them.

CARS VERSUS PEOPLE

When matched against a motor vehicle, people usually lose. More than 8,000 pedestrians die every year in the U.S. in the traditional match-up of man versus machine. Although this is the highest number of pedestrian deaths in the world, it is not the highest rate when compared to total population. That distinction goes to Hungary; Yugoslavia and West Germany share second place.

Near Joplin, Missouri, on June 25, 1946, a bus hit a cow and crashed, killing twelve passengers.

Most pedestrian fatalities occur in the early afternoon and early evening. Friday is the deadliest day. Crossing at an intersection is fatal to about a quarter of the total; another 30 percent of these ill-fated walkers die while crossing between intersections.

In 1958, twenty-eight children were killed when their school bus ran off the road in Prestonburg, Kentucky, and fell fifty feet into a river.

CARS VERSUS BICYCLES

The number of bicycles in the U.S. has been increasing at a dramatic rate, but in recent years the fatality count has remained fairly steady. The U.S.

averages more than 1,000 deaths per year for bicycle riders, with about 1.2 deaths per 100,000 bicyclists. Until 1972, bicycle deaths most commonly involved children — as many as 75 percent of the total fatalities were under the age of fourteen. Since the bicycle craze caught on with teenagers and adults in the early 1970s, this rate has changed. Deaths are now more equitably distributed among all age groups, with children gaining most from the change — less than 35 percent of all bicycle fatalities now come from this group.

A minor traffic accident proved lethal for a motorcycle rider in Japan. Upon collision, his ballpoint pen punctured his body, causing death.

TREES VERSUS AUTOMOBILES

About 100 people are killed every year in the U.S. from collisions between vehicles and animals.

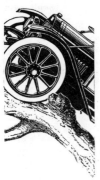

Trees are not generally considered an enemy of mankind. However, when a moving vehicle takes on a tree, the tree usually wins. According to one safety expert, "We find that trees are the number one offender among deadly fixed objects when ranked by accident severity."

About 3,000 automobile fatalities occur each year in which a tree is the primary destructive agent. Because of the compact, immovable mass that a tree represents to a moving vehicle, the impact between them is almost always more severe than when the other objects are other vehicles, walls, or barriers. The energy represented by the moving vehicle cannot be partially dissipated by deflection or absorption when the object it strikes is as concentrated and rooted to the spot as a tree. Consequently, if a vehicle does strike a tree, severe damage to the vehicle and its passengers can occur at much lower speeds than when the impact is with another type of object.

Studies have shown that the average speed of vehicles that collide with trees when fatalities occurred is 31.5 miles-per-hour. However, because of the severity of the impact, fatalities have resulted when speeds were as low as 15 miles per hour (the passengers were not using seat belts). In fact, damage and injury is so much more severe when the object involved is a tree that local officials typically overestimate the speed of impact by at least 100 percent in more than half of the accidents they investigate.

At any speed in excess of 25 miles per hour, fatalities are likely to occur to any unrestrained passenger. If the passengers are using restraints, including shoulder harnesses and seat belts, their chances of surviving a collision when their vehicle exceeds 35 miles per hour is still considered uncertain, at best.

Every year, there are about 13,000 automobile accidents with fixed objects that result in fatalities. Of this number, 3,000 fatalities result from impacts with trees, and 1,500 from impacts with utility poles. Using average figures, one out of every ninety-five drivers will be involved in an accident with a tree (not necessarily resulting in death) during a driving career. Most of these collisions will occur on undivided two-lane roads, on a curve in more than half the cases. About 85 percent of the people killed by trees are male, and half of them are between fifteen and twenty-four years old. Half of the fatalities involve alcohol, and at least 95 percent of the deceased do not wear any kind of restraining device.

Although it is obvious that driver error is the primary cause of the fatalities in most of these cases, a lack of signs and road indicators — especially

Travelling abroad can be deadly — an average of twenty Americans die every year while outside the country.

Since 1940, at least forty jockeys have died from accidents while racing horses.

The automobile is the most deadly object available to the average consumer according to fatality statistics, followed by cigarettes, then alcohol.

The first death from a motor vehicle accident in the world was on August 17, 1896, near the Crystal Palace in London, England. A car giving demonstrations ran over a panic-stricken onlooker, Mrs. Bridget Driscoll, and crushed her skull.

where there are curves — is often a contributing factor. Even drunk drivers could do a little better at negotiating road hazards if the hazards were adequately marked. However, the removal of potentially hazardous trees everywhere they are found could be an impossible task — one study of two states in 1974 estimated that 5 to 8 million trees were in dangerous locations.

Most deadly state: **Vermont** (18 percent fatality rate).

Least deadly state: **Nevada** (1 percent fatality rate).

_____TRAINS VERSUS CARS

For as long as trains have crossed roads, people have been getting killed at these crossings. Most railroad crossing deaths occur because of a lack of caution on the part of motorists, although relatively few actually result from a complete lack of warning barriers.

These sample figures indicate how crossing fatalities happen: in 1980, 708 people died while in their vehicles; of this total, 75 percent of the vehicles were struck by a train and 25 percent ran into a train. A total of ninety-two people were killed in vehicles that ignored or drove around crossing gates, including four fatalities from vehicles that actually stopped before proceeding onto the crossing. Only three fatalities occurred at crossings with no signs or signals of any kind.

Forty-one percent of the fatalities occurred at night (not including dusk), and 54 percent during daylight hours (not including dawn). The weather was rarely a factor — 65 percent of all these

Candidate for most bizarre transportation accident: a passenger train on the Hudson River Railroad ran into a river schooner in 1851 with an unrecorded number of fatalities. The ship had been blown onto shore and upended on the railroad tracks, where the train, running in heavy fog, hit it.

accidents in 1980 occurred in clear weather conditions, 8 percent in the rain, 3 percent in the snow, and 2 percent in fog.

When Auto Fatalities Occur:

Most deadly hour	**4:00 to 5:00** P.M.
Least deadly hour	**4:00 to 5:00** A.M.
Most deadly day	**Saturday**
Least deadly day	**Sunday**
Most deadly month	**February**
Least deadly month	**April**

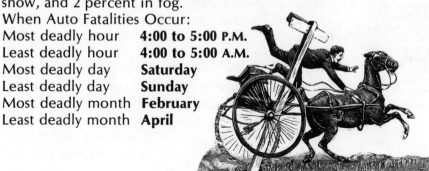

MILITARY JEEP DEATHS

"We may suppose that the final aim of the destructive instinct is to reduce living things to an inorganic state. For this reason we call it the death instinct."
— Sigmund Freud

A test of late-model cars in 1984 by the Department of Transportation indicated that almost half of the vehicles would not prevent fatal injuries to occupants from crashes at 35 miles per hour.

Drivers of military jeeps are involved in more than their share of traffic accidents, and oftentimes deaths result. In one two-year period (1979-1981), there was a total of sixty-four military deaths associated with jeep accidents. This total included fifty-four fatalities in Army jeeps, eight in Marine jeeps, one in an Air Force jeep, and one in a Navy jeep.

The high accident rate for military jeeps (there was a total of 2,847 accidents reported in this same two-year period) has been blamed mostly on stability problems with the vehicles on roads. Because they are designed for off-the-road use, they do not respond in predictable ways when

On June 11, 1955, two race cars in the Le Mans Grand Prix in Le Mans, France, crashed, then careened into a crowd of spectators; eighty-three people died.

The worst railroad accident in the world was in Modane, France, on December 12, 1917; 543 people died in the wreck.

The first American railroad fatality was on June 17, 1831. An engine fireman was killed by an exploding boiler in a locomotive in South Carolina.

The worst railroad accident in U.S. history was in Nashville, Tennessee, on July 9, 1918; there were 101 deaths.

driven on paved surfaces by personnel accustomed to the handling characteristics of commercial vehicles. Only a very small percentage of these accidents have been attributed to vehicle failures, but alcohol was involved in at least 120 of the accidents reported.

If the number of fatalities is compared to the number of accidents for each branch of the service separately, there are some interesting differences. The highest percentage of fatalities occurred with the Marine jeeps, where 7 percent of the 121 accidents involved deaths. The Army rated a distant second, with 2 percent of its 2,472 accidents involving deaths. Both the Air Force and Navy scored the lowest fatality index, with 1 percent of their total accidents involving deaths (133 accidents with Air Force jeeps, 121 accidents with Navy jeeps).

_____CASEY JONES, YOU BETTER WATCH YOUR SPEED

"Let us hope that when we are dead
things will be better arranged."
— Marcel Proust

Many train travelers choose that mode of travel out of a fear of flying. However, trains are not necessarily guaranteed to get everyone to every destination without injury. Some of the worst disasters in the nation's history have been on the rails.

Just as with airplanes, defective equipment and bad judgements by the operating personnel are usually the causes of accidents. Similarly, both kinds of transportation provide little protection for passengers when a crash occurs. In the case of trains, there are usually more survivors for any given wreck. While a plane crash is almost certain to kill most of those on board, there are a few train accidents with more than 100 fatalities.

Before railroad tracks were made in one piece, the rails were made of wood with an iron strip fastened to the top. These strips were known to spring up and spear themselves through the floors of passing railroad coaches, often with gruesome, and fatal, results for the passengers.

Safest rail month **May**
Most deadly month **August**
Most deadly state **New York**

Train wrecks with large loss of life (U.S. only):

		Fatalities
Ashtabula, Ohio	December 29, 1876	92
Chatsworth, Illinois	August 10, 1887	81
Atlantic City, New Jersey	July 30, 1896	60
Eden, Colorado	August 7, 1904	96
Wellington, Washington	March 1, 1910	96
Ivanhoe, Indiana	June 22, 1918	68
Nashville, Tennessee	July 9, 1918	101
Brooklyn, New York	November 2, 1918	97
Philadelphia, Pennsylvania	September 6, 1943	79
Rennert, North Carolina	December 16, 1943	72
Richmond Hill, New York	November 22, 1950	79
Woodbridge, New Jersey	February 6, 1951	84

In 1944, a train stalled in a tunnel in Salerno, Italy; 426 people died from asphyxiation.

OPEN BRIDGES

☐ May 6, 1853: 46 people died when a New Haven Railroad train drove onto an open drawbridge at Norwalk, Connecticut.

☐ October 28, 1906: 57 people died when a Pennsylvania Railroad train drove onto an open drawbridge at Atlantic City, New Jersey.

☐ September 15, 1958: 48 people died when a Jersey Central train drove onto an open drawbridge at Newark Bay.

A drawbridge collapsed with a train on it, drowning thirteen people in Oakland, California, in 1890.

WINGS VERSUS RAILS

Francis Gary Powers, who survived being shot down in a CIA spy plane over the U.S.S.R., later lost his life in a helicopter accident in Los Angeles, California, while flying a media mission for a local television station.

Despite the gruesome consequences for those involved in railroad wrecks, train travel is about the safest way to change locations, given the total number of miles involved. In 1980, there were 11 billion total miles traveled by passengers — and four deaths. The only other form of mass transportation that is safer is scheduled airlines (as separate from private airplane travel), which had 221 billion total miles of passenger travel in 1980 — and eleven passenger deaths. The comparison: 0.04 passenger deaths per 100,000,000 passenger miles on trains versus 0.01 passenger deaths per 100,000,000 passenger miles on airplanes.

Because one accident on either an airplane or a train can drastically alter the death rate for the whole year, it is interesting to compare the two forms of transportation in past years.

On September 17, 1908, Thomas Selfridge, a lieutenant in the U.S. Signal Corps, became the first person to die in an airplane crash, when a plane piloted by Orville Wright with Selfridge as an observer crashed in Fort Meyer, Florida. Wright escaped death, but sustained injuries.

| | RAILROAD | | AIRLINE | |
	Fatalities	Rate	Fatalities	Rate
1965	12	.07	205	.38
1970	10	.09	0	.00
1975	8	.08	113	.08
1980	4	.04	11	.01

The final results from this 20-year period: trains were safer (less lethal) for eleven years, airplanes were safer for seven years, and for two years both methods tied.

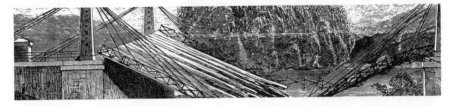

THE ICARUS SYNDROME

"The god-men say when die go sky
Through Pearly Gates where river flow,
The god-men say when die we fly
Just like eagle-hawk and crow —
Might be, might be; but I don't know."
— Australian Aborigine Saying

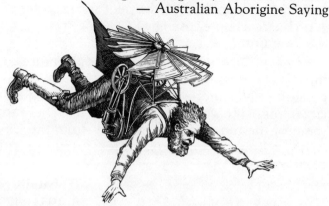

Orville Wright, co-inventor of the airplane, died of natural causes at the age of seventy-six in Dayton, Ohio, on January 30, 1948. On the same day, three separate U.S. airplane crashes left fifty people dead.

Almost as early as man took to the air, he began plummeting to the earth, the victim of gravity and aviation accidents. However, with the advent of modern technology and public pressure to improve safety, the safety record of flying machines has improved dramatically.

Most aviation accidents today involve private airplanes — about 1,500 fatalities annually. Although weather conditions account for some of these, the major cause of most is pilot error. In recent years, there have been about forty deaths a year from helicopter accidents, not including military or commercial flights. With the rapidly expanding use of helicopters by television stations, these media copters have begun to gain a share of

When airplanes were still a novel invention, seat belts for pilots were installed only after the consequence of their absence was observed to be fatal — several pilots fell to their deaths while flying upside down.

these problems. Included in the copter disaster hall of fame:

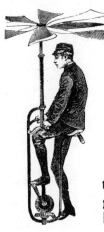

☐ Francis Gary Powers, the former pilot of a U-2 spy plane shot down over Russia, was killed when his copter crashed in Los Angeles in 1977, during a TV news-gathering mission.

☐ In Dallas, Texas, in 1980, three members of the WFAA-TV news team died in the crash of their copter.

☐ In Colorado, in 1982, the pilot and reporter on board a copter used by KCNC-TV crashed, killing both.

However, it is the spectacular misadventures of the larger passenger airplanes that hold the greatest public interest, because of the subsequent larger loss of life when an accident occurs. These are some of the most notable examples from the U.S. (with a few foreign examples included for comparison):

			Fatalities
Tokyo, Japan	U.S. Air Force	June 18, 1953	129
The Grand Canyon	Two airliners collide	June 30, 1956	128
New York City	Two airliners collide	Dec. 16, 1960	134
Paris, France	Air France jet	June 3, 1962	130
Maracaibo, Venezuela	Venezuelan airliner	Mar. 16, 1969	155
Toronto, Canada	Canadian airliner	July 5, 1970	109
Morioka, Japan	Japanese jet and fighter	July 30, 1971	162
Moscow, U.S.S.R.	Russian airliner	Oct. 13, 1972	176
Miami, Florida	Eastern Airlines	Dec. 30, 1972	101
Paris, France	Turkish airliner	Mar. 3, 1974	346
New York City	Eastern Airlines	June 24, 1975	113
Canary Islands	Pan Am — KLM ground collision	Mar. 27, 1977	582
San Diego, California	Commercial — private plane collision	Sep. 25, 1978	144
Chicago, Illinois	American Airlines	May 26, 1979	272

WHEN TO WORRY

Most accidents and resulting fatalities on airlines occur during approaches and landings. The next most dangerous period is during take-off. The two categories combined account for more than 70 percent of all airline deaths. The safest time in the air is the period between take-off and landing, when there is only equipment malfunction, collision with other planes, and terrorism to worry about. Through the end of the 1970s, terrorism accounted for about 5 percent of all fatalities; 25 percent were caused by malfunction and collision.

The most dangerous airlines in the world:

ALIA	(Royal Jordanian Airlines)
THY	(Turkish Airlines)
AVIACO	(Spain)
TAROM	(Rumanian Airline).

Two Air France planes — on separate flights from Saigon to Paris — crashed in the same area near Bahrain in the Persian Gulf on June 12, 1950. Forty-seven people died in one crash; forty in the other.

Parachustists have a favorite term for the results of a chute failure; they call it "buying a farm."

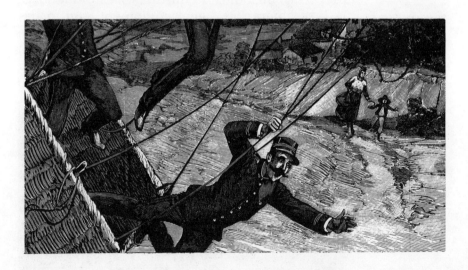

DOWN WITH THE SHIP

*"Man with the burning soul
Has but an hour of breath
To build a ship of truth
On which his soul may sail —
Sail on the sea of death,
For death takes toll
Of beauty, courage, youth,
Of all but truth."*
— John Masefield

In nearly sixty years (from 1788 to 1847) of slave trade, 22 percent died en route from Africa to the Americas, according to a report in a French journal from the period. Of a total of 1,462,000 slaves, 327,000 died aboard slave ships.

One thousand fishermen drown every year in the U.S.

An escalator in a subway station in Moscow collapsed on February 19, 1982, killing fifteen people.

Of all forms of transportation, water-born transportation has one of the most dismal records for safety. Even in recent times, when technology and safety methods exist to protect vessels and passengers, needless fatalities occur. However, in the premier days of sail, when there was no alternative to ocean travel, there were many other problems, including a consistent lack of lifeboats, lack of emergency signal equipment, and inadequate navigational devices. These added to the immense toll of ships and human life that the sea took each year. In the mid-1800s, the loss of life from British ships alone was more than 4,500 annually.

The ferocity of the oceans and waterways of the world and the carelessness with which man has traversed them have provided a never-ending supply of bones for Davey Jones's Locker. The final toll from shipping accidents, as well as can be estimated, is probably more than 1,000,000 lives since the first intrepid native sailor drowned in a dugout.

Since the Air Force was organized in 1947, there have been five accidents in which civilian and Air Force planes have collided.

Some of the notable losses on the seas and rivers:

	Ship		Fatalities
English coast	*Royal George*	August 29, 1782	900
Mississippi River	*Sultana*	April 27, 1865	1,547
East River, New York	*General Sloc*	June 15, 1904	1,021
Atlantic Ocean	*Titanic*	April 15, 1912	1,513
St. Lawrence River	*Empress of Ireland*	May 29, 1914	1,024
Chicago River	*Eastland*	July 24, 1915	812
Baltic Sea	*Gustoff Wilhelm*	January 30, 1945	8,000
Japan	*Ferry*	September 26, 1954	1,172
Java Sea	*Tamponas II*	January 27, 1981	580

—FAMOUS PEOPLE WHO DIED IN TRANSPORTATION ACCIDENTS

In 1970, fifty-two injured passengers from a train accident in Nigeria were killed when the truck carrying them to a hospital crashed.

Airplane crashes: Knute Rockne, Will Rogers, Carole Lombard, Glenn Miller, Dag Hammarskjold, Buddy Holly, Michael Todd, Otis Redding, Rocky Marciano, Roberto Clemente, Jim Croce, Dolly (Mrs.) Sinatra, Audie Murphy, Thurman Munson

Automobile wrecks: General George Patton, Jackson Pollack, Albert Camus, Jayne Mansfield, Margaret Mitchell, Grace Kelly, James Dean

"The statistics of suicide show that, for non-combatants at least, life is more interesting in war than in peace."
— W. R. Inge

Chapter Five

BY THEIR OWN HAND
Death by Suicide and Self-Destruction

As far as we know, suicide is a peculiarly human act; there is no evidence that any other species of the animal kingdom willfully enacts self-destruction.

In the U.S., suicide is officially listed as the tenth leading cause of death. It accounts for more than 25,000 fatalities annually (according to the most recent statistics available). Suicide statistics, however, are more unreliable than those for other causes of death; the actual figure could easily be as much as twice the official count. If this is the case, then suicide would claim the fourth position among leading causes of death in the U.S., surpassed only by heart disease, cancer, and accidents.

Suicide has existed in all cultures since the beginning of recorded history. In most cultures, suicide has been generally regarded as anti-social behavior — except in certain situations among the privileged classes, most notably, when it was offered as a means of execution.

The Christian religion regards self-destruction an impious act. To both Catholics and Moslems, it is an abhorrent act, and the devout of both religions exhibit a comparatively low suicide rate in comparison with members of other religious groups.

Suicides among both the young and the terminally ill have increased in the U.S. since 1950. While suicide is no longer a crime in any state, helping someone commit suicide is considered either murder or manslaughter in most states.

Since about 1960, firearms have been the most common method of suicide. About 65 percent of male suicides use this method while only about 35 percent of female suicides prefer it. Poisoning — which includes drug overdoses, liquids, and gasses — ranks second overall as the method of suicide, but first among women as the favored method. Prior to 1960, hanging was the second most common means, but it now ranks a poor third.

A seasonal peak in suicides occurs during the spring months. Winter is generally the low season, although a slight increase takes place around the Christmas holidays. According to one researcher, people of slight physique tend to commit suicide in early spring, and those who are stockier, toward the end of spring.

Frankie Lymon, lead singer with the Teenagers, died in 1968 from an overdose of heroin in his grandmother's bathroom in New York City.

Donnie Hathaway, singer and arranger, committed suicide in 1979 by jumping off the roof of the Essex House Hotel in New York City.

Virginia Woolf killed herself in 1941 by placing a heavy rock in the pocket of her coat and walking into the River Ouse in England.

NOTABLE SUICIDES

Some of the famous people from history who have taken their own lives include:
Socrates, Nero, Cleopatra, Romeo and Juliet, Samson, Saul, Judas, Marilyn Monroe, Judy Garland, Jim Jones, Ernest Hemingway, Carole Landis, Christopher Marlowe, Brian Epstein, Virginia Woolf, Tim Hardin, and Richard Brautigan.

SUICIDE IN THE U.S.

Method	Male 1960	Male 1980	Female 1960	Female 1980
Firearms	7,879	12,937	1,138	2,459
Percent of Total	54.2	63.1	25.3	38.6
Poison	2,631	2,997	1,699	2,456
Hanging/Strangulation	2,576	2,997	790	694
Other	1,453	1,574	875	755
TOTAL	14,539	20,505	4,502	6,364

	Total Male And Female 1960	Total Male And Female 1980
Firearms	9,017	15,396
Percent of Total	39.8	57.7
Poison	4,330	5,453
Hanging/Strangulation	3,366	3,691
Other	2,328	2,329
TOTAL	19,041	26,669

SUICIDE AROUND THE U.S.

"However great a man's fear of life . . . suicide remains the courageous act, the clear-headed act of a mathematician. The suicide has judged by the laws of chance — so many odds against one, that to live will be more miserable than to die. His sense of mathematics is greater than his sense of survival."
— Graham Greene

Where you live apparently has some influence on your likelihood to commit suicide. For instance, the Rocky Mountain region had the highest suicide rate, 16.2, while New England was the region with the lowest, 9.5 for the year 1980.

Highest suicide rate   **Nevada** (22.9)
Lowest suicide rate   **New Jersey** (7.4)
National average (1980)   **11.9**
Honorable mention — states with rates close to the
top   **Alaska, Arizona**

Hart Crane, a popular writer, committed suicide on April 27, 1932, by jumping over the side of a ship off the coast of Mexico.

_____SUICIDE FACTS

"We only die when we fail to take root in others."
— Leon Trotsky

SUICIDES INCREASE WHEN
☐ Unemployment is high
☐ Public figures commit suicide
☐ Entertainers die
☐ Television characters commit suicide
☐ Divorce rate increases
☐ There are low death rates for other causes
☐ A nation is at peace
☐ Population is at low density

During World War I, suicide rates dropped in Europe in both those countries involved in the fighting and those that were neutral. Following the armistice, the rates began to return to pre-war levels.

SUICIDES DECREASE WHEN
☐ Wars occur
☐ Population is at high density
☐ Unemployment is low
☐ Divorce rates decrease
☐ Death rates from other causes are high

Spring is the deadliest time of the year for suicides, and winter, the least deadly.

Here's what we do know about suicide in the U.S.:
☐ People kill themselves more often than they kill others.
☐ Suicide is more prevalent among the elderly than among the middle-aged or the young.
☐ Men commit suicide at almost THREE TIMES the rate of women.

Only 10 to 15 percent of all suicide victims leave notes, making the determination of cause of death much easier. Most will reveal some kind of verbal clue as to their intentions before a suicide attempt. Generally, victims suffer from various states of depression before an attempt is made.

□ Women attempt suicide THREE TIMES as often as men.

□ Firearms are the most common means of suicide among males.

□ Drugs are the most common means among females.

□ High-risk categories include policemen, soldiers, mental patients, drug addicts, students, alcoholics, and the elderly.

□ Factors that indicate a low potential for suicide include: female gender, youth, rural occupation, religious devoutness, marriage, large number of children, membership in lower socio-economic classes.

□ The suicide rate seems to vary inversely with the homicide rate.

□ Suicide is extremely rare among young people under the age of fifteen, but the suicide rate in the fifteen to twenty-four age group is growing rapidly in most modern countries.

□ The suicide rate in the U.S. appears to be increasing, while all other causes of death are showing a gradual decrease.

There seems to be a global geographical correlation: northerly places, such as Scandinavia, show higher suicide rates than more tropical climates.

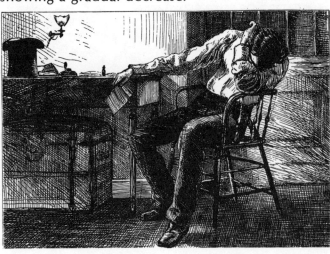

They don't call it "Stormy Monday" for nothing — and "Tuesday's just as bad." According to suicide statistics, Monday is the favored day for self-destruction. In 1979, (an average year), about 82 suicides occurred nationwide every Monday. Saturday statistics, by contrast, showed an average of 71 suicides, the lowest rate among days of the week.

One study concludes that 75 percent of all automotive accidents with only a single vehicle involved could be suicides.

SUICIDE RATES (U.S.A., 1980)

	MALE		FEMALE		TOTAL	
	White	Black	White	Black	White	Black
5-14	.7	.3	.2	.1	.5	.2
15-24	21.4	12.3	4.6	2.3	13.1	8.9
25-34	25.6	21.8	7.5	4.1	17.1	16.0
35-44	23.5	15.6	9.1	4.6	16.3	10.5
45-54	24.2	12.0	10.2	2.8	17.8	8.0
55-64	25.8	11.7	9.1	2.3	18.4	8.5
65 and over	37.5	11.4	6.5	1.4	23.3	7.7
All Ages	19.9	10.3	5.9	2.2	13.3	7.2

TOTAL POPULATION

	Rate
5-14	.4
15-24	11.0
25-34	16.6
35-44	13.4
45-54	12.9
55-64	13.5
65 and over	15.5
All Ages	10.3

LOOK BEFORE YOU LEAP

The Golden Gate Bridge, considered the number one choice in the world for suicides — more more than 750 have occurred since its opening in

1937 — doesn't deliver all of its victims into the water. As many as 25 percent of the leapers off this span leap before they look, and die crashing into the ground, or the roofs of buildings of the U.S. military base that lies under the San Francisco side. The Officer's Mess, which was the final destination for some of these bodies, was finally moved to a new location after a few too many meals were disturbed by these uninvited guests.

William Hall, an Englishman, killed himself in 1971 by boring eight holes into his head with an electric drill.

ALARMING DEADLY TREND

"A suicide kills two people, Maggie, that's what it's for!"
— Arthur Miller

Religion has an influence on suicide rates. Predominantly Catholic countries, where suicide is considered a mortal sin, seem to show reduced rates.

In the past twenty-five years, the U.S. suicide rate among the young has increased dramatically. The rate, which began to increase in the mid-1950s, had more than tripled for the fifteen to twenty-four age group by 1978. Suicide was the fifth leading cause of death for this age group in 1950, but became the third leading cause before 1980. (Vehicular fatalities are the primary cause of death for this age group. Homicide ranks second — except among blacks where homicide is the leading cause of death among fifteen to twenty-four-year-olds.)

Women who have attempted or committed suicide during the premenstrual period are much more likely to have been living with a man, than to have lived alone.

Between 1970 and 1978, the suicide rate for fifteen to twenty-four-year-olds increased 41 percent: 39,011 U.S. residents in this age group committed suicide. The suicide rate for this group went from 8.8 per 100,000 population to 12.4 per 100,000 between 1970 and 1978, while the rate for the remainder of the population remained stable.

This rate increase was due primarily to the 47.4 percent rise among male suicide victims, from 13.5 to 19.9. The female increase over the same period was only 11.9 percent, from a rate of 4.2 to 4.7. Therefore, by 1978, the suicide rate among males of this age group was four times that of females. Additionally, it was only among white males that such a significant increase occurred; the rate among non-white males showed only a gradual increase.

Norman Morrison, a Quaker, died in 1965 from burns suffered after he set himself afire outside the Pentagon office window of Defense Secretary Robert McNamara — a protest against U.S. involvement in Vietnam.

Most of the suicides for this age group actually occurred among the young adult population — twenty to twenty-four-years-old — accounting for more than twice as many suicides as the adolescent ages of fifteen to nineteen. A significantly higher rate exists for adolescents in the western states than for the rest of the country.

James Forrestal, former Secretary of Defense of the U.S., died after leaping from the 16th floor window of the National Naval Medical Center in Bethesda, Maryland.

During these three decades, the method of suicide also changed for all races and both sexes in this age group. The use of firearms and explosives increased, and poisoning, the traditional method among women, showed a corresponding decrease.

Among the fifteen to nineteen age group, the suicide rate more than doubled between 1960 and 1980 and is now the third leading cause of death. From a rate of 5.2 in 1960, the suicide rate has increased to 12.5 by 1980 for this age group. Among college students, it is the second leading cause of death.

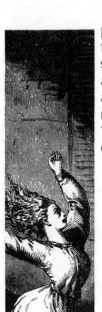

At the height of popularity for ritual suicide (hari-kari) in Japan, many people killed themselves after victory was declared in the war with China (1895). This was not to celebrate, but to protest the leniency of the peace terms.

One researcher places the number of attempted suicides in this age group at half-a-million annually. This would mean that fifty-seven adolescents attempt suicide every hour throughout the U.S.

Psychologists have postulated possible reasons for this suicide increase among the young. They include: greater acceptance of violence both in the family and the society, tendency of parents to spend less time with their children, the dissolution of the family, and cultural frustration described generally as loss — loss of family love, loss of control over their own destiny, loss of identity, loss of self-worth, and the loss of meaning in life.

Persons older than sixty-five (11.3 percent of the population — 25.5 million in 1980) account for one-fourth of all suicides. In 1980, while the national suicide rate was 11.9 for all ages, for the sixty-five and older age group it was 35 percent for males and about 6.1 percent for females, giving a combined rate for the age group of thirty-one deaths per 100,000 population, about 25 percent of all suicides committed.

SOAPY SUICIDES

A study conducted in 1982 found that suicides in the U.S. tended to increase following any episode on a television soap opera in which a suicide was attempted or committed. Although the results of this study are subject to other possible influences, suicide prevention centers report that there are increased number of calls to suicide "hotlines" following these episodes, plus anytime there is an actual suicide reported of a popular television or movie star. In the U.S., hero-worship can literally be a way of life and death.

WORLDWIDE SUICIDE SURVEY

"If one denies that there are grounds for suicide one cannot claim them for murder. One cannot be a part-time nihilist."
— Albert Camus

Worldwide, more than 100,000 people die by their own hands every year. The motives and methods of suicide victims vary greatly, as do contemporary cultural attitudes toward it.

Suicide cases are cited in our earliest cultural history. Samson killed himself, Saul fell on his sword, and Judas hanged himself. The Jews committed collective suicide rather than renounce their faith to either the Romans or the Crusaders. In ancient times, it was considered admirable among some cultures for virgins to kill themselves to preserve their virtue. Some religious sects even condoned suicide as a means of warding off sin.

Although contemporary attitudes toward suicide are generally more tolerant than in the past, most cultures and religions regard suicide as an abomination. The Jewish, Christian, and Moslem religions are among the most stringent in their attitudes toward self-destruction. The *Koran*, for example, decries suicide as an act worse than homicide.

In western culture, from the time of the ancient Greeks until the Renaissance, most societies condemned suicide except when committed by members of the privileged classes. Although Pythagoras and Plato abhorred the act, the Greek tragedies elevated it to an act of sacrifice among the royalty.

A recent study concluded that almost 40 percent of all suicides in prison are committed within the first two weeks of incarceration.

A report by an insurance research group in the early 1980s indicated that more than 80 percent of the drivers in a test sample of auto crash fatalities had one or more drugs in their systems. The drivers who had taken drugs were almost always at fault in the cause of the fatal accidents.

Among occupations, physicians have one of the highest suicide rates. Suicide claims more than 25 percent of all deaths for doctors under the age of forty, with the preferred method being hanging.

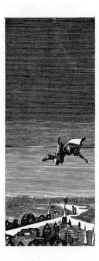

To the Romans, the suicide of a slave was regarded as a theft, since it represented a loss of property; a Roman soldier who survived a suicide attempt was executed, since it represented an act of desertion.

In the Christian Europe of the Middle Ages, suicide was regarded as an act of Satan. Corpses were mutilated, refused burial in the church cemetery, and had their property confiscated. Until about 150 years ago, suicide victims in Britain were buried at a crossroads with a stake through their hearts.

Among the most famous instances of ritual suicide is the *sepeku*, a compulsory disembowlment, which could be ordered of a vassal by any feudal chief in Japan, until it was outlawed in 1868. This practice still occasionally occurs today. World War II kamikaze bombers evolved from this cultural milieu.

The Hindu practice of *Sattee*, which required a widow to immolate herself on her husband's funeral pyre, was finally outlawed by the British, after a rash of 2,000 such suicides occurred in India in 1821. Occasional reports indicate this tradition hasn't completely expired.

The assault on the Jewish fortress of Massada — in which all inhabitants committed suicide rather than be captured — and the recent episode of mass suicide instigated by the Reverend Jim Jones in Jonestown, Guyana, represent the most monumental acts of self-destruction recorded in history.

More recently, there has developed among religious and nationalist fanatics a predilection for suicidal acts of terrorism; suicide bombers, for instance, have been increasing in number. With an increase in religious or nationalistic fanaticism, there seems to be a corresponding increase in this destructive form of suicide.

A good contemporary example is the Shiite Muslim suicide bombers. Their zeal to die in a *Jihad*, or holy war, thus assuring themselves of a passport to heaven, is a convenience not many military tacticians enjoy. If they take a large number of infidels with them, so much the better. But — one expert on the *Koran* says there is nothing in it that states killing is a passport to heaven.

A popular song was written following the suicide leap by Billie Joe McAllister off the Tallahatchee Bridge in Mississippi on June 3, 1953.

WORLDWIDE SUICIDE DEATH RATES

HIGHEST	DEATH RATE (per 100,000)
Hungary	43.1
Austria	23.8
Switzerland	24.1

LOWEST	
Nicaragua	0.9
Philippines	0.8
Egypt	0.1

(The U.S. ranks twelfth worldwide: 11.9 suicides per 100,000 population.)

There were twenty-five known deaths from participation in the game of "Russian Roulette" after the movie *The Deer Hunter* was first shown on television.

_____SUICIDAL GENIUS

In one of the more unique prison suicides ever recorded, William Kogut, a San Quentin inmate sentenced to be executed for murder, blew himself up on October 9, 1930. Even though prison officials had carefully removed everything they could to prevent him harming himself before the state could do its duty, he made an ingenious pipe bomb. By scraping the red spots off of a deck of playing cards, and filling a hollow bed leg with these explosive dots, he created a destructive weapon. The bomb was detonated with the heat from the heater in his cell, after he had placed his head on top of it.

POSSIBLE SUICIDE DEATHS

"It's not that I'm afraid to die. I just don't want to be there when it happens."
— Woody Allen

In the margin:

In 1933, fifty-six children jumped more than 1,000 feet to their deaths from the edge of the crater of the Mihara Volcano on the island of Oshima in Japan. Police guards were eventually assigned to prevent any more jumps.

The popular game "Dungeons and Dragons" has been implicated in the motivation for at least nine suicides and murders, according to one survey.

The disparity between the official body count and the possible count of suicide victims exists for a number of reasons. Generally, suicide is listed as a cause of death only if the circumstances unequivocally warrant such a determination: when a suicide note is left by the victim of sudden death, when the victim has a history of suicidal tendencies, or when the cause of death could be nothing but suicide.

In the absence of such obvious clues, most officials are reluctant to rule a death a suicide. In fact, shoptalk amongst coroners indicates that in many small communities, suicides are rarely listed as such on death certificates. Often, this is the only practical thing for a coroner to do, when the pressures of life in a small community dictate unwritten rules of conduct. Many coroners are also the personal physicians for the community, and can rarely afford to jeopardize their income by antagonizing their clients.

Any number of traffic fatalities, especially those involving one person and a stationary object, could very likely be impulsive suicides. At least one estimate suggests that 75 percent of all such accidents are suicides; however, there is no way to prove such a theory. The same theory could also be applied to alcohol abuse, drug overdoses, firearm

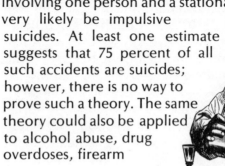

accidents, or even violent behavior that results in a homicide or death from legal intervention. A conservative interpretation of this approach would put the actual number of suicides at twice the official figure.

Additionally, numerous forms of self-destructive behavior that eventually result in accidental death or in demise due to chronic health problems are often long-term suicides — people who have been killing themselves over a period of time. They are never listed as suicides. Victims of such determined self-abuse are more likely to be listed among the mortality statistics for heart disease, pneumonia, cirrhosis of the liver, or accidental death under any one of numerous categories: drug overdose, drowning, auto accident, fire, pneumonia, falls, misadventure, poisoning, and hanging.

A book was published in France in 1982 that described in detail how to commit suicide. Within a few months, the book sold enough copies to be on the best-seller list in that country, and at least ten suicides were directly attributed to it.

Normally the following are likely to be suicides: Hanging, self-immolation, cut throat, crushing under a train, and car exhaust poisoning.

The following are regarded as problematic: Fall from a height, drowning, firearms, poisoning, and drug overdose.

Almost certainly accidental: Fall on a level surface and multiple vehicle traffic accident.

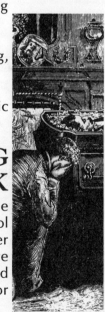

DROWNING IN DRINK

A study from 1972 shows that almost half of the drowning victims included in a survey had alcohol in their blood when they died. Results from other studies showed even higher numbers, up to a figure of 69 percent. In thirty fatalities involving spas and hot tubs since 1979, twelve listed alcohol as a factor in the death — 40 percent of the total.

DRUG ABUSE

"If this is dying, I don't think much of it."
— Lytton Strachey

Drug overdoses claim about 7,000 lives in the U.S. annually. As in the past, 75 percent or more of these fatalities are caused by legally prescribed drugs; less than 25 percent are caused by illicit drugs.

In 1982, a retired businessman in Kentucky invented a self-serve method for funerals. He drove to a mortuary, left a list of funeral instructions with the receptionist, and then shot himself in the parking lot.

U.S. DRUG OVERDOSE DEATHS

	Illegal Drugs	Legal Drugs	Total
1980	1,242	3,535	4,777
1981	1,367	3,888	5,255
1982	1,735	4,046	5,781
1983*	1,843	4,515	6,358
1984*	1,993	5,001	6,994

(* Projected)

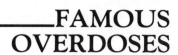

FAMOUS OVERDOSES

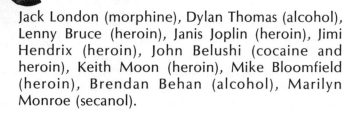

Jack London (morphine), Dylan Thomas (alcohol), Lenny Bruce (heroin), Janis Joplin (heroin), Jimi Hendrix (heroin), John Belushi (cocaine and heroin), Keith Moon (heroin), Mike Bloomfield (heroin), Brendan Behan (alcohol), Marilyn Monroe (secanol).

HIGH-CLASS DOPE DEATHS

"Account ye no man happy till he die."
— Euripides

Although heroin use in the United States is primarily concentrated among low-income urban dwellers, there has been a noticeable increase in recent years in the use of heroin by the middle class. With this increase has come higher rates of overdose and death.

Drug counselors, doctors, and experts on drug use all agree that there is a new and growing popularity for this illegal and addictive drug. While its prevalence continues in low-income urban areas, it is finding fashionable new acceptance with professionals, business executives, and others of the middle class who claim to find it useful in "leveling off" the over-stimulation that can come with cocaine usage. It is believed by those observers close to the problem that this usage will continue to increase, as will the number of deaths from overdose, the misuse of drugs in combinations, and the related illness and disease associated with improper injections and unclean equipment.

One sure result from such a problem in America's clean middle-class ranks will be action taken and money spent to control the use of these drugs, and to rehabilitate those who have become addicted to them. The use of heroin by those on the bottom rungs of society has been largely ignored, as they have no real power and their loss of life has been traditionally overlooked. But when voters and taxpayers suffer from the same problem, the wheels will turn swiftly to alleviate the suffering.

Until recently, it was extremely rare to find fatalities from overdoses of cocaine. Epidemic use of this illicit drug is now resulting in such cases in increasing numbers.

A recent study of mice indicates that increased sexual activity is related to shortened lifespans, at least in mice.

_____DEAD DRUNK

"Some of us may die.
Remember, statistically
It is not likely to be you.
All flags are flying fully dressed
On government buildings — the sun is shining
Death is the least we have to fear."
— Peter Porter

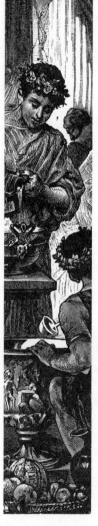

From the beginning of written history, it has been recorded that death has resulted from the excessive consumption of alcohol. In addition to fatalities directly attributable to alcohol abuse, chronic health problems indirectly contribute to the death of the habitual drinker. But social customs and societal acceptance of heavy drinking have changed. Consider the changing quantities of alcohol consumed in the U.S.:

1800	6.6 gallons per person (of drinking age) per year
1850	2.1
1900	2.0
1950	2.0
1970	2.4
1980	2.8

These drinking patterns closely parallel changes in mortality rates from alcohol-related diseases. Some earlier sources attributed deaths directly to alcoholism, but then, as now, fatalities described as cirrhosis are often actually the result of excessive alcohol consumption. One early 1900's report listing alcoholism as a cause of death specified that twice as many women died from it as men.

An examination of fatality rates from cirrhosis of the liver is accepted by some medical authorities as a relatively acceptable method for tracking alcohol abuse. In fact, studies comparing these rates with alcohol consumption show that fatalities will climb when more alcohol is consumed, and decline when less is consumed. During the era of prohibition in the U.S., there was a marked drop in the death rate from cirrhosis, indicating that the reduced flow of liquor was a help to the general health of the nation. Of course, during Prohibition, the influx of illegally manufactured alcohol that contained poisonous materials added to the overall mortality rate by killing some of the people who drank it.

Homemade liquor killed 100 revelers at a wedding in New Delhi, India, in 1972.

Thirty-nine people — all black — died and many others were blinded for life after drinking an improperly prepared batch of bootleg whiskey in Atlanta, Georgia in 1951. Another group of twenty-five drinkers died in New York in 1928 after drinking a batch of illegal brew made from denatured alcohol.

OLD-FASHIONED DRINKING PROBLEMS

An official report from England in 1896 showed these results for those who died from drinking, out of a sample of hundreds:
1 Ploughman, 2 gardeners, 3 printers, 3 cotton-spinners, 3 cutlers, 4 carpenters, 4 shoemakers, 4 fishermen, 4 miners, 5 stonecutters, 6 farmers, 8 blacksmiths, 8 drapers, 10 grocers, 11 tailors, 12 painters, 15 bakers, 19 costermongers, 23 butchers, 23 commercial travellers, 25 brewers, 33 cab drivers, 55 publicans.

The same source listed the years of drinking required to end in death:

For women	14 years
gentlemen	15 years
working classes	18 years
Drinking beer	22 years
spirits	17 years
mixed	16 years

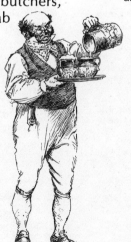

RED, DRUNK, AND DEAD

The U.S.S.R. has the highest mortality rate in the world for alcohol-related deaths. Its average annual death rate for alcohol poisoning is twenty deaths per 100,000 population, ten times higher than the average for other countries. Many of these deaths are attributed to homemade brews, which often contain impurities or alcohol levels in excess of commercial brands.

SEX DEATHS

"The goal of all life is death."
— Sigmund Freud

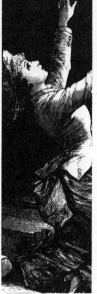

Terry Kath, a member of the rock group Chicago, died in 1978 while trying to prove a gun wasn't loaded — by pointing it at his head and pulling the trigger.

Even to the enlightened and liberal minds of the modern world, some of the beliefs and understandings of past generations appear strange and unthinkable, if not altogether absurd. One of these concepts, the belief that masturbation was a harmful disease, was not just popular folklore, but a widespread doctrine in the medical community through the 1800s.

Scientists and doctors thought that the achievement of orgasm through self-stimulation involved different processes in the body than did intercourse, and was not only a sinful activity, but dangerous to the health of an individual. It was commonly believed that masturbation caused dyspepsia, epilepsy, blindness, impotency, loss of memory, rickets, consumption, insanity, and general debility. Some reports and studies emphasized that excessive masturbation could cause death.

Although no complete analysis is available for

such statistics, at least one hospital record from the period lists fatalities from this sexual problem. An eighty-six-year record from the Charity Hospital of Louisiana in New Orleans indicates for posterity that one patient died in 1872 and one in 1887, both from masturbation. A third death in 1888 was attributed to anemia brought on by masturbation.

A hospital report from the late 1800s listed several patient deaths from masturbation.

Currently, masturbatory behavior can be unhealthy in some cases. Many men have been known to die accidentally while attempting to achieve a sexual climax during controlled strangulation. This method of sexual stimulation involves a belt or cord around the neck that is suspended over an elevated object. Despite the inherent dangers, many devotees think that this kind of strangulation will not lead to death, as fainting will cause the hold on the cord to loosen and permit normal respiration.

Felix Faure, the president of France in 1899, died from a heart attack while in bed with his mistress.

Unfortunately, there are numerous cases where circumstances keep this from happening, and a dead body results — left in a questionable and tell-tale position. Although some of these cases are officially classified as suicide, the technical label for the practice is autoerotic asphyxia, and in Los Angeles County alone, officials estimate there are twenty to thirty deaths a year from the practice. Nationwide, there are an estimated 500 to 1,000 deaths a year.

Leo VIII, pope of the Catholic Church in 965 A.D., died of a stroke while committing adultery.

The Federal Bureau of Investigation, which has examined some of these fatalities, believes that most victims of this "crime" are male, with an average age of twenty-six. One expert on this phenomena believes there are thousands of practitioners in the U.S.

*"Unusual irritability, which leads to
quarrels, shortens life."*
— St. Thomas Aquinas

Chapter Six

BY ANOTHER'S HAND
Death by Murder and Legal Intervention

Homicide is the killing of one person by another. Distinctions between different types of homicides vary according to traditions, cultures, and legal systems. In the U.S., homicides may consist of the following:

Murder. The intentional killing of another person.

Manslaughter/Criminal Negligence. The death of an individual brought about unintentionally through carelessness or neglect of another.

Legal Intervention. The death of an individual brought about by an agent of the judiciary in the line of duty. Generally refers to killing by a law enforcement officer in the line of duty.

Execution. The enactment of a capital punishment sentence imposed by civilian or military judicial authority.

Combat Fatalities. Death brought about through military conflict.

Assassination. The murder of a public figure, especially a political figure.

Infanticide. The murder of a newborn infant.

Patricide. The murder of a father by his progeny.

Matricide. The murder of a mother by her progeny.
Justifiable Homicide. The killing of another under justifiable circumstances, such as self-defense.

In 1980, 24,278 homicides occurred in the U.S. This constituted a death rate of 10.7 per 100,000 population, which made homicide the eleventh leading cause of death in the U.S. About 50 percent of these killings were perpetrated with handguns, of which there were 11 million in the U.S. at the time. An additional 12 percent of these deaths were caused by other kinds of firearms.

Taken together, the 13,650 homicide victims killed by firearms, the 15,396 suicides committed with firearms, and the 1,955 fatal accidents involving firearms in 1980, put the total U.S. firearm body count for the year at 31,001.

In the thirty-year period between 1950 and 1980, the murder rate in the U.S. more than doubled, going from 5.3 per 100,000 population to 10.7. The number of murder victims in that period tripled from 7,942, to 24,278.

The 1980 death rate for white males was 10.9, and for white females 3.2. Black males had a death rate of 66.6, and black females, 13.5. Murder victims for that year included 114 infants, and 165 law enforcement officers.

When he was a boy, Juan Carlos, the current king of Spain, accidentally shot and killed his younger brother with an air-rifle.

According to a study in 1973, there were fewer murders on sunny days than on cloudy days, indicating that psychological effects from weather conditions may play an important part in society.

Most likely victims   **Black males**
Most deadly region   **The South** (14.7 per 100,000)
Least deadly region   **New England** (3.8 per 100,000)
Most deadly state   **Alaska** (18.5 per 100,000)

U.S. MURDER PROBABILITY

Edward "Blackbeard the Pirate" Teach, died near Ocracoke Island, North Carolina, on November 21, 1718, during an intense struggle in which he had been shot five times and cut twenty-five times by a cutlass. The fight ended when someone hit him from behind with a sword, severing his head.

"Love cannot be much younger than the lust for murder."
— Sigmund Freud

The possibility that you will be murdered is present throughout your lifetime, but the chances vary with sex, race, and age. The lifetime chance of a U.S. citizen becoming a murder victim is 1 in 153.

For males specifically, the probability is 1 in 100, while for females, it is 1 in 323. Non-white races have a greater probability than whites. For both males and females, those between the ages twenty and thirty constitute the most murder-prone age group. A steady decline occurs from age thirty on. For younger ages, under twelve, the chances of being murdered are greatest at infancy, and lowest between the ages of five and twelve.

Here's the grim breakdown, according to the U.S. Department of Justice:

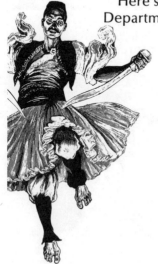

Classification	Odds
U.S. Total	1 in 153
Male	1 in 100
Female	1 in 323
White Total	1 in 240
Male	1 in 164
Female	1 in 450
Non-White Total	1 in 47
Male	1 in 28
Female	1 in 117

MOTIVES

"Nobody dies nowadays of fatal truths:
There are too many antidotes to them."
— Friedrich Nietzsche

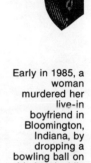

About 55 percent of all murders are committed by a relative or acquaintance of the victim. Arguments result in 42 percent of these killings. Seventeen percent of the murders are within family relationships, and half of these involve spouse killing spouse. Here's a four-year comparison:

	1977	1980
Total	18,033	21,860
Percent	100.0	100.0
Felony Total	16.7	17.7
Robbery	9.9	10.8
Narcotics	1.7	1.7
Sex Offense	1.7	1.5
Other Felony	3.4	3.7
Suspected Felony	5.9	6.7
Argument Total	46.6	44.6
Romantic Triangle	2.8	2.3
Alcohol/Narcotics	5.3	4.8
Property/Money	3.3	2.6
Other Arguments	35.2	35.0
Other Motives/Circumstances	16.6	115.9
Unknown Motives	14.2	15.1

Early in 1985, a woman murdered her live-in boyfriend in Bloomington, Indiana, by dropping a bowling ball on his head while he slept.

WHAT A WAY TO GO

Roy Sullivan, a retired park ranger, died from a handgun wound (possibly self-inflicted) to the head on September 28, 1983. It seems odd that a mere gun accomplished what one of nature's deadliest forces had failed to do — Sullivan is listed in the *Guinness Book of World Records* as the "lightning conductor of Virginia," after being struck by lightning seven times in his life and surviving each strike.

Alaska is the deadliest state in the U.S. for murders, with a rate of 18.5 murders per 100,000 people; North Dakota has the lowest rate, with 0.7 murders per 100,000.

WEAPONS

"After life's fitful fever, he sleeps well;
Treason has done his worst: nor steel nor poison,
Malice domestic, foreign levy, nothing
Can touch him further."
— Shakespeare

As recently as the early 1980s, killing was involved in the activities of almost two out of every ten leading characters on television. At the same time, the stereotyped murder victims remained old women, poor women, and black women.

Firearms are far and away Americans' favorite weapons for doing each other in. Here are the facts for 1980's carnage:

Weapon	Number Of Victims	Percent
Firearms	13,650	62
Handguns	10,930	50
All Others	2,720	12
Cutting/Stabbing	4,212	19
Blunt Object	1,094	.05
Strangulation/Beating	1,666	.08
Arson	291	.01
All Others	947	.04
Total	**21,860**	**100**

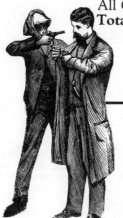

WORLDWIDE MURDER RATES

"The scorn of death is again one of the methods of prolonging life . . . The best way not to die too soon is to cultivate the duties of life and the scorn of death."
— St. Thomas Aquinas

The prevailing notion that modern Western societies are more violent than traditional cultures and developing nations is not reflected in a comparison of international homicide rates (see below). Theories linking the crime rate to the stress of urban life, unemployment, overcrowding, and diminished family ties also appear to be refuted by the data.

Many countries with high murder rates are rural societies. The incredible murder rate for top-of-the-list Lesotho is attributed to tribal tensions, rivalries, and vendettas — primarily over the theft of livestock. It is interesting to note that none of the top ten countries on the homicide list appear in the statistics elsewhere in this book, charting cancer, heart disease, and suicide death rates.

Data presented here covers the mid-1970s and was published by INTERPOL, in *International Crime Statistics*.

DEADLIEST COUNTRIES	DEATH RATE (per 100,000)
Lesotho	140.81
Bahamas	22.88
Guyana	22.21
SAFEST COUNTRIES	
Greece	0.87
Spain	0.67
Norway	0.50

(The U.S. is eleventh in rank in the world: 10.7 homicides per 100,000 population.)
Note: Executions are excluded from the category of homicide, but the separate governments define other categories differently.

SEE NO EVIL

Max Geller, the owner of the Green Parrot Bar in New York City, was shot and killed during an apparent robbery on July 12, 1942. None of the

If all of the gunfights, bushwackings, murders, duels, and feuds from the era of the Old West (roughly 1850 to 1900) are included, the total number of people killed by bullets during that time was about 20,000.

twenty customers in the bar at the time admitted seeing the shooting. A police detective studied the case for several years and finally identified the culprit with the help of the bar's resident parrot. The bird just kept repeating the name of the murderer until someone listened to him.

U.S. MURDER RATES
(per 100,000 population)

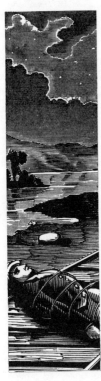

MOST DEADLY STATES		LEAST DEADLY STATES	
1. Alaska	18.5	1. North Dakota	0.7
2. Texas	16.1	2. Nebraska	2.0
3. Louisiana	16.0	3. Maine	2.1
4. Mississippi	14.0	4. New Hampshire	2.2
5. Nevada	13.6	5. Iowa	2.3

MURDER FACTS

"Virtue and vice are the only things in this world, which, with our souls, are capable of surviving death."
— Ethan Allen

□ One third of the prison inmates convicted of murder were under the influence of drugs, alcohol, or both at the time of their crime.

□ Women constitute 13 percent of all homicide arrests.

□ One quarter of all inmates in U.S. penal institutions are convicted of murder or manslaughter.

□ More than half of all homicides are committed by someone known to the victim.
□ Seventeen percent of all homicides are committed by relatives of the victim.
□ Half of all murders are committed with handguns.
□ Since 1900, more Americans have been murdered with handguns than the number of American servicemen who have died in all foreign wars.
□ A murder is committed every twenty-three minutes in the U.S.

Murder charges were filed against a mother in California for the death of her seven-year-son — in order to discipline him she had forced him to eat more than four pounds of food at one sitting.

—ASSASSINATIONS IN THE U.S.

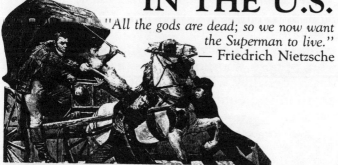

"All the gods are dead; so we now want the Superman to live."
— Friedrich Nietzsche

Mrs. Lucinda Mills, age sixty seven, was strangled to death in 1933 by her family during a religious ceremony inside her home near Tomahawk, Kentucky.

Abraham Lincoln, President of the U.S. April 14, 1865.
James Garfield, President of the U.S. July 2, 1881.
Carter H. Harrison, Mayor of Chicago. October 28, 1893.
William Goebel, Governor of Kentucky. January 30, 1900.
William McKinley, President of the U.S. September 6, 1901.
Anton J. Cermak, Mayor of Chicago. February 15, 1933.
Huey P. Long, U.S. Senator from Louisiana. September 8, 1935.
Medgar Evers, Field Secretary of the N.A.A.C.P. June 12, 1963.
John F. Kennedy, President of the U.S. November 22, 1963.
Malcolm X, religious leader. February 21, 1965.

Reverend Martin Luther King, religious leader. April 4, 1968.
Robert F. Kennedy, U.S. Senator from New York. June 5, 1968.
Cleo A. Noel, U.S. Ambassador to the Sudan. March 2, 1973.
George C. Moore, U.S. Charge d'Affaires. March 2, 1973.
Rodger P. Davies, U.S. Ambassador to Cyprus. August 19, 1974.
Col. Paul R. Shaffer, U.S. representative in Iran. May 21, 1975.
Lt. Col. John H. Turner, U.S. representative in Iran. May 21, 1975.

___DEATH PENALTY

Several dogs, four calves, and a horse were electrocuted on March 2, 1889, to demonstrate the effectiveness of electricity for executions.

"If you put me to death in spite of my declared innocence, you will do me less harm than you do yourselves."
— Socrates

The death penalty has been a reality since the beginnings of history. However, it has been more common in "civilized" societies than in tribal ones. In the U.S., ironically enough, the majority of those who oppose abortion and euthanasia favor the death penalty, while most of those who favor abortion and euthanasia are opposed to the death penalty.

Mary, a circus elephant, was charged with the deaths of three men, and lynched in Tennessee. The lynching — which took place in Erwin, Tennessee, on September 13, 1916 — was accomplished with a steel cable attached to a railroad derrick after two unsuccessful attempts. More than 5,000 people watched.

In ancient and medieval times, the death penalty was enacted for a wide variety of offenses, many of which were trivial. Methods of execution were also numerous and quite cruel in many cases. The most common form of execution, hanging, was originally used primarily for the lower classes. (During the reign of Henry VIII in England, 65,000 public hangings took place. Beheading was usually reserved for the nobility, usually in private.)

Until this century, public execution of criminals was commonplace because governments considered it a deterrent for the populace to witness enactments of the death penalty. The last public execution in the U.S. was in 1936 when 20,000 people gathered in Owensboro, Kentucky, to witness the hanging of a black man, Rainey Bethea, for the murder of an elderly white woman. The last public execution in France took place in 1939 when convicted murderer Eugene Weidmann was beheaded at the Palace of Justice, Versailles.

During the reign of Queen Mary of England in the sixteenth century, she became known as "Bloody Mary" for her large-scale executions of non-catholics; as many as 300 heretics were burned at the stake while she ruled the country.

THE EXECUTIONER'S SUM

"To circumvent death, to evade it, is one of the oldest and strongest desires of rulers."
— Elias Canetti

In 1547, English law was ammended to end the practice of boiling people to death as punishment for certain types of criminal behavior.

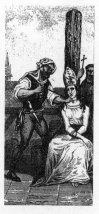

With Supreme Court challenges to statutory death penalties pending, no executions occurred in the U.S. between 1967 and 1976. Then came Gary Gilmore. The moratorium on executions ended on January 17, 1977, when Gilmore faced a Utah firing squad.

Between 1930 and 1967, 3,862 civil executions took place in the U.S.; an additional 160 were carried out by the military. The majority of the civil death penalties were imposed on black men.

CIVIL EXECUTIONS IN U.S. (1930-1981)

	White	Black	Total
1930-1939	827	816	1,667
1940-1949	490	781	1,284
1950-1959	336	376	717
1960-1967	8	2	10
1968-1976	---	---	---
1977-1981	4	---	4
Total	**1,754**	**2,066**	**3,862**

Offense			
Murder	1,667	1,630	3,337
Rape	48	405	455
Others	39	31	70

The only execution of a war criminal from the Civil War was carried out on November 10, 1865. The criminal, Henry Wirz, had been in charge of the Andersonville prison in Georgia during the war. When sentenced, he said, "I'm damned if the Yankee eagle hasn't turned out to be what I expected, a damned turkey buzzard."

During the reign of terror after the French Revolution, a condemned man who was a friend of the executioner arranged to signal after the guillotine had severed his head to demonstrate "life after death." The executioner reported that he saw his friend wink after the blade had performed its function.

ABOUT FACE

"There is no confessor like unto Death!
Thou canst not see him, but he is near:
Thou needst not whisper above thy breath,
And he will hear."
— Henry Wadsworth Longfellow

On June 20, 1864, in Petersburg, Virginia, during the American Civil War, the Union Army hung a black man after convicting him of raping a white woman. The hanging was performed in view of Confederate forces, who were expected to be impressed with the North's ability to carry out justice. However, the opposite effect was accomplished, as the southern army made sure that its black workers understood that they would also be hanged if they tried to escape to the other side. Before the hanging, hundreds of blacks had escaped; afterwards, for a period of weeks, none crossed the dividing line.

CAPITAL PUNISHMENT ILLEGAL

*"In the last analysis, it is our conception
of death which decides our answers to all
the questions that life puts to us."*
— Dag Hammarskjold

The death penalty has been abolished in seventy-three countries worldwide. Portugal was the first, voiding its capital punishment laws in 1867. Holland followed suit (except for certain military offenses) in 1870. Then came Norway (1902) and Sweden (1921). Ireland abolished the death penalty in 1964; England, in 1965; Bolivia, in 1966. Except for treason, there has not been a death penalty in either Italy or Switzerland for many years. The Soviet Union abolished capital punishment after World War II, but reinstated it in 1950.

In the U.S., forty-one states allow capital punishment. The death penalty is off the books in these states:
Michigan (1847), Wisconsin (1853), Maine (1887), Minnesota (1911), Alaska (1957), Hawaii (1957), Oregon (1964), Iowa (1965), and West Virginia (1965).

Other states have abolished capital punishment except in special circumstances. In 1852, for example, Rhode Island disallowed death as a punishment for all criminals except those who murder while serving a life sentence. Other states that have similar laws are New York, Vermont, New Mexico, and North Dakota.

British law was changed in 1790 to stop the execution of women by burning; thereafter those women sentenced to death would be hanged, instead. The last woman to be burned was Christian Bowman, who was executed on March 18, 1789, for making counterfeit coins.

A "hangman's wages,' according to a published report from London in 1813, were about seven shillings, with another four shillings to be paid for the stripping of the body.

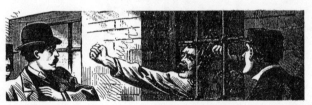

THE FIRST TO FRY

On September 30, 1630, John Billington became the first person to be executed in America. He was hanged for murder, having shot and killed an antagonist during an argument.

The first person executed in the electric chair had a gruesome experience as a human guinea pig. William Kemmler, an ax murderer, was electrocuted on August 6, 1890, in Auburn Prison in New York. The first jolt, lasting seventeen seconds, failed to kill him. A second, seventy-second jolt succeeded not only in killing Kemmler, but also in making some of the witnesses nauseous as they watched his body being literally cooked to death. An observer at the autopsy observed that his flesh resembled well-cooked beef, and that the excess current had carbonized some of the muscles.

On October 15, 1917, Mata Hari, exotic dancer and convicted spy, was executed by a firing squad in Vincennes, France. Twelve members of the firing squad, plus an officer, fired at her. However, an autopsy revealed only four bullets in her body.

LYNCHING

"O death, where is thy sting? O grave, where is thy victory?"
— I Corinthians, XV: 54

Lynching is generally defined as the unlawful killing of a person by a mob, generally by hanging, and usually associated with vigilante justice and racial violence. The term is believed to have originated from the actions of Captain William Lynch, who was known for his acts of violence against the British during the Revolutionary War in Virginia. Or, it can be traced to a justice of the peace in Virginia named Judge Charles Lynch, who, during the same period, was known for dispensing justice — particularly in the form of flogging people known to be loyal to the Crown — without due process of law.

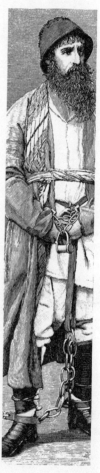

The last public lynching in the U.S. is generally believed to have been in 1946 when two black men and two black women were hanged in Walton County, Georgia. The last known non-public lynching involved a black serviceman who was hanged in August, 1982; this lynching also took place in Walton County, Georgia. Although the local coroner's office ruled this incident a suicide, civic groups from the area believe lynching was the cause of death.

Hanging has not always been the preferred method of execution in lynchings. In one ten-year period alone (1918-1928), 10 percent of the reported instances of lynching used fire. Victims in these cases were burned alive, and even some of the unfortunates who were hanged were also burned after they were cut down. In this same period, beating and dismembering were also used in a few cases.

Although the South has won the undisputed title of "Lynching Capital of the U.S.," it is not the only place where this method of justice has been used. In fact, there are only a few states where no lynchings have ever been recorded — but there is no way of determining if this is just because of a lack of reporting. In addition, although most of the known lynchings are of black people, there have also been hundreds of whites and Asians who were lynched. The final toll for a few western states indicates that more whites than blacks have been lynched.

LYNCHING

	White	Black	Total
1885	110	74	184
1890	11	85	96
1895	66	113	179
1900	9	106	115
1905	5	57	62
1910	9	67	76
1915	13	56	69
1920	8	53	61
1925	0	17	17
1930	1	20	21
1935	2	18	20
1940	1	4	5
1945	0	1	1

More than 1,000 criminals have been executed in the electric chair since its introduction in the U.S. in 1890.

The last execution with a guillotine took place in France on May 12, 1973.

Philip Spencer claims the dubious distinction of being the only U.S. Naval officer ever to be executed for mutiny. Along with two enlisted men, he was hanged on December 1, 1842, on a return voyage from Africa on the USS *Somers.* A postmortem court martial acquitted Spencer of the mutiny charges.

Total includes years between dates shown above. *Note: A total of 4,751 lynchings have been verified by research from the Tuskegee Institute and Walter White; a separate figure by the N.A.A.C.P. in 1928 listed a total of 4,950 lynchings since 1882.*

The researchers who compiled these figures also reached some interesting conclusions. In a group of states from the South with the highest numbers of lynchings, it was discovered that the fewer residents there were in a county, the greater the number of lynchings. It was also discovered that women were not excluded as victims of this exclusive club — ninety-two were lynched between 1882 and 1927.

MOST DEADLY STATES (1882-1956)

	White	Black	Total
Mississippi	40	537	577
Georgia	39	491	530
Texas	141	352	493
Louisiana	56	335	391
Alabama	48	299	347

LEAST DEADLY STATES (1882-1956)

	White	Black	Total
District of Columbia	0	0	0
Connecticut	1	0	1
Maine	1	0	1
New Jersey	0	1	1
Delaware	0	1	1

Constitutional Rights Hall of Fame (no reported lynchings in these states): **Massachusetts, New Hampshire, Rhode Island, Vermont**.
Constitutional Rights Hall of Shame (highest number of lynchings in the U.S.): **Mississippi, Georgia, Texas**.

——DECAPITATIONS

"I shall never act differently, even if I have to die for it many times."
— Socrates

The most infamous means of execution by decapitation is, of course, the French guillotine. During the French Revolution, thousands of the aristocracy were dispatched beyond the pale. Prior to this clever invention, however, decapitation was an ever-popular means of execution, especially for the nobility. Thousands of victims from virtually all cultures have lost their heads on the executioner's block. But a sharp axe blade and steady hand were no match for Mr. Guillotine's clever invention.

The following notables from history all lost their heads, the result of political ill-health:
John the Baptist, Saint Paul, Saint Alban,
Saint George, Anne Boleyn, Lady Jane Grey,
Mary, Queen of Scots, Earl of Essex,

The last public lynching in the U.S. took place in 1946 in Walton County, Georgia, when two black men and two black women were hanged.

More whites than blacks have been lynched in Indiana, Iowa, Kansas, Montana, Nebraska, New Mexico, Oklahoma, South Dakota, and Wyoming.

Between 1882 and 1927, ninety-two women are known to have been lynched in the U.S.

Sir Walter Raleigh, Charles I, Duke of Monmouth, Louis XVI, Marie Antoinette, Maximilian Robespierre, Prince Faisal, Sir Thomas More, and the statue of the Little Mermaid (later restored).

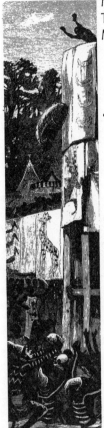

INFANTICIDE

". . . But in truth, love conquers nothing — certainly not death — certainly not chance."
— Archibald Macleish

Infanticide — killing the newborn — has been widely practiced in most cultures since prehistoric times. It still occurs in the active form — abrupt termination of the infant's life — and in the passive form — where neglect and inattention eventually result in the infant's death. Vestiges of this practice are referred to in contemporary American culture as "child abuse."

Since most cultures cherish their progeny, tolerance of this seemingly contradictory practice is ascribed to various motives. Religious sacrifice, especially of the firstborn, is described in Hebrew scriptures, and in the histories of Egypt, Greece, and Rome. Such ritual infanticide, which continued in India until the nineteenth century, represented an offering to the deity of one's most valuable possession.

Some societies practiced infanticide as a means of ridding themselves of weak and deformed children. Others engaged in the practice to destroy defective offspring, or to eliminate questionable offspring, such as births resulting from incest, rape, or conceived out of wedlock.

Anthropologists maintain that female infanticide was the primary means of population control in most parts of the world until the twentieth century. Recently, accusations have been made that this practice is still widespread in China because of government policies.

Infanticide was common among western cultures through classical times. Christian Emperor Constantine outlawed infanticide in the fourth century, and it remains a crime in most parts of the world today.

Ironically, Christian Europe's zeal to wipe out baby killing had quite the opposite effect. In fact, concurrent Christian policies of executing mothers responsible for infanticide, while supporting male feudal prerogatives and condemning childbirth out of wedlock, was probably responsible for baby-killing in larger numbers than at any other time in history.

Most young women of the lower classes preferred execution to the pious persecution of unwed mothers and the onus of illegitimacy for their bastard offspring. Yet, to be at the disposal of the master's or employer's sexual appetites was one of the services a servant or peasant woman was often required to render.

This kind of victimization of young women was responsible for countless unwanted pregnancies and subsequent suicides. Members of the military exercised a similar prerogative, which together with rape, accounted for more unwanted pregnancies.

As successive waves of disease and famine engulfed Europe over the next few centuries, many young women found prostitution their only means to avoid starvation, causing still more unwanted pregnancies and infant deaths.

And finally, another means emerged by which an enterprising young woman might gain employment

During a wave of anti-Chinese sentiment in the U.S. in 1880, Henry Ward Beecher said, "We have clubbed them, stoned them, burned their houses and murdered some of them; yet they refuse to be converted. I do not any way, except to blow them up with nitroglycerin, if we are ever to get them to Heaven."

Giles Cory was the last person to be pressed to death as punishment for a crime in the American colonies. He was executed in 1692 in Salem, Massachusetts. In England, pressing was continued until 1726.

Many animals have been executed throughout history, usually for crimes associated with sorcery or witchcraft. Recorded instances of animal punishment include cases involving birds, pigs, insects, wolves, and a cow that was hanged in France in 1740.

and avoid hunger — that is, by becoming a wet nurse in the home of a patrician family. Such employment was plentiful and honorable and persisted until the development of bottled formula in this century.

Unfortunately, this convenient service provided to the upper classes promoted infanticide, since offering this service first required childbirth. It was extremely rare, however, for a wet nurse to have children of her own.

Throughout these centuries, women bore sole responsibility for such unwanted pregnancies and the ensuing infanticides. In Europe during the Middle Ages, conviction for infanticide often involved execution by drowning —the mother was usually sewn into a sack with a cat, a dog, and a snake, then submerged for six hours.

Just how many infants perished and mothers were executed during this period is impossible to determine. Best guesses range in the hundreds of thousands.

In 1386, a pig killed a young child in Europe. Popular belief at that time held that the devil controlled the pig. The swine was subsequently dressed in men's clothing and executed.

ABORTIONS

"Of all the benefits virtue confers on us, the contempt of death is one of the greatest."
— Michel de Montaigne

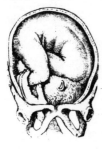

The abortion is the most common operation performed in the U.S. Since the legalization of abortion in 1973, more than 15 million women have undergone this procedure. Most abortions are requested by unmarried white women: about 70 percent of these women are white and about 75 percent are unmarried.

LEGAL ABORTIONS

1973	615,873	1979	1,251,921
1974	763,476	1980	1,553,890
1975	854,853	1981	1,631,595
1976	988,267	1982	1,713,970
1977	1,079,430	1983	1,798,875
1978	1,157,776	1984	1,888,770

In the largest execution in U.S. history, thirty-eight Sioux Indians were hanged in Mankato, Minnesota, on December 23, 1862.

——OUTFLANKED

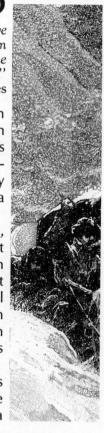

"And now the time has come when we must depart: I to my death, you to go on living. But which of us is going to the better fate is unknown to all except God."
— Socrates

The consumption of human flesh, although generally frowned upon in polite society, has been a fairly common practice by several diverse groups throughout history. Anthropophagy, as cannibalism is known, is usually either a ritualistic ceremony or a religious phenomenon. It can also be a desperate act of survival.

The Aztecs, in ceremonies at hundreds of temples, killed and totally or partially consumed at least 15,000 sacrificial victims annually. In the South Pacific, raids by meat-seeking island tribes might have also accounted for similar numbers of annual fatalities. Records from the island of Fiji confirm that, over the years, the practice of cannibalism expanded until extraordinary quantities of humans were devoured.

In these and other examples, cannibalism was often associated with an appreciation for the taste of human flesh. In other instances and cultures, a

Every seventeen minutes, a firearm kills somebody in the U.S.

More than 68,000 men died in the 99-year history of "Devil's Island," the French penal colony in the Cayenne Islands. It was officially closed by the French government in 1938, but hundreds of prisoners died there after that date because of the lack of transportation home due to the intervention of World War II.

Thirteen prisoners died while attempting to escape from Alcatraz prison in San Francisco Bay during its 29-year history, from 1934 to 1963.

taste for one's fellow man was not the motivation for killing and eating humans. Instead, all or part of the bodies were consumed as a final ritual of victory over a conquered foe.

The noteworthy occurrences of this anti-social behavior in Western civilization are most often associated with matters of survival. The most recent example is the well-publicized plight of the Uruguayan rugby team who were stranded in the Andes Mountains after a plane crash. Those players who died in the crash provided nourishment for the survivors.

Another celebrated cannibalism case involved the infamous Alferd Packer. Stranded in the Colorado Rockies in 1874, Mr. Packer ate five members of his traveling party. Packer achieved notoriety as much from the identity of the victims as from his method of disposing of them. The judge who tried his case had special cause for vengeance: Packer's companions comprised the majority of Democrats in the county. The judge condemned the cannibal with these words: "There was seven Democrats in Hinsdale County, and you've ate five of them, God damn you. I sentence you to be hanged by the neck until you is dead, dead, dead, as a warning against reducing the Democrat population of the state. Packer, you Republican cannibal, I would sentence you to hell but the Statutes forbid it." Although found guilty, Packer escaped execution because of a legal technicality.

The rugby team and Packer do not represent isolated experiences. Particularly common on the high seas, cannibalism often occurred among sailors set adrift in small boats in the aftermath of ship sinkings. In a precedent-setting example, two English sailors were found guilty in 1884 of killing and eating a shipmate in order to survive while adrift at sea. Many similar incidents took place during an era when rescue at sea was the exception rather than the rule.

In many, if not most of these cases, the survivors who consumed their fellow passengers also pre-arranged the availability of the bodies. In other words, humans killed humans for food. Records show that in some instances, group decisions involved either lots being drawn or volunteers being requested. Some evidence suggests that before such decisions were made, choices occasionally might have been weighed in favor of the hungriest.

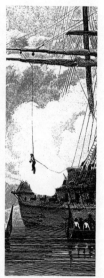

___POISONED PENS

"Fortune awaits the aspiring scribe with many wiles, and oft treats him sorely."
— P. H. Ditchfield

It has often been said that the pen is mightier than the sword. History also shows that the pen can be fatal to its user as well. Since the first written word, the editorial view of the author has been arousing ire of readers, and in not a few instances, this has led to the extinguishing of that view permanently. The following are some notable examples:

Antonio de Dominis, Archbishop of Spalatro, published several books, but he made a fatal error with one that claimed that the Holy Scriptures proved that the Bishop of Rome had no authority. Although he lived in England, he was tricked into moving to the continent, where he was imprisoned by the Inquisition, and died. After his body had been burned, a colleague described him: "He was a malcontent knave when he fled from us, a railing

In India, a caste of criminals known as Thugs preyed on travelers for six centuries until they were suppressed in the 1800s by the British. They developed their murder and robbery techniques in the religious service of a special group of gods, and considered their victims to be sacrifices.

knave when he lived with you, and a motley parti-colored knave now he is come again."

John Biddle, an early Unitarian, died in prison in 1662, the victim of his opinion, which was expressed in a book entitled *The Faith of one God, who is only the Father, and of one Mediator between God and man, who is only the man Christ Jesus; and of one Holy Spirit, the gift, and sent of God, asserted and defended in several tracts contained in this volume.*

Urban Grandier, clergyman and author, wrote a book advocating marriage for the clergy, and was later burned at the stake in Loudon, France, for supposedly casting spells on the nuns at a convent.

Lucilio Vanini, an Italian philosopher, was burned alive at Toulouse in 1619. The Inquisition disagreed with a book he had written that attempted to prove atheism invalid; their opinion was that he had not done a very good job.

Antonius Palearius, an Italian professor, was either beheaded, hanged, strangled, or burnt to death, according to various sources, in the mid-1500s. His crime was publishing a book attacking the Inquisition — which pronounced sentence upon him for refusing to sign his name by crossing the "t," the sign of the cross.

John Fisher, the bishop of Rochester, was beheaded at the request of King Henry VIII of England on July 22, 1535. He had written a work critical of the King's divorce. His last words were, "Feet, do your duty; you have only a short journey."

Algernon Sidney, an English author, was beheaded in 1683 for treasonous opinions. A manuscript found in his house was used to condemn him. An excerpt from it said, "Liberty is the mother of virtues, and slavery the mother of vices."

Trajan Boccalini, an Italian writer, was the victim

Harry Robbins, a murderer who was sentenced to the electric chair in New York State, agreed to try to wiggle his fingers as he was being electrocuted. The experiment was designed to see how quickly this method of execution worked. When the switch was pulled, no movement was observed.

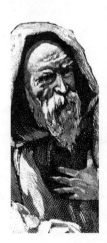

of his satire on the Spanish rulers in Italy about 1615. In Venice, he was beaten to death by hired assassins wielding bags of sand.

Cecco d'Ascoli, an Italian poet and professor of astrology, was burned alive in Bologna in 1327, after casting an unpleasant horoscope for a local Duke.

Nicodemus Frischlin, a German poet, died from injuries received when a rope made from bedclothes broke as he was escaping from prison in the late 1500s.

Caspar Weiser, a professor in Sweden, was beheaded in 1676 because of a single verse he wrote welcoming the victory of the Danish army. The Danes were expelled shortly after by the Swedish army, with the poem and author left behind to their fate.

John Williams, an English poet, was hanged and drawn and quartered in 1619 because of a poem foretelling the early death of King James.

Pierre Petit, an unpublished poet who lived in Paris, was hanged and burned during the middle of the seventeenth century. A priest discovered one of his poems that had been blown out of the window by the wind, and raised a stink which resulted in the poet's sudden demise. The subject of the poem was supposedly scandalous.

And finally, there's an exception to this list, a writer who escaped his destiny. **Theodore Reinking**, a Swedish historian, wrote himself into jail with a book in 1644. After years of imprisonment, he was offered the choice of either losing his head or eating his words. The author opted for the latter; it is recorded that he escaped death by concocting a sauce from his book, and dining on his own words.

High murder rates are not confined to urban societies; the highest death rate for murders in the world is in Lesotho, in South Africa, with 140 murders per 100,000 people.

For three days in July, 1863, riots in New York City caused the deaths of over 1,000 people. This civil violence was partly instigated by U.S. government draft laws, but mostly involved with racial hatred between Irish immigrants and blacks.

_____RIOT DEATHS

"He not busy being born
Is busy dying."
— Bob Dylan

A piano tuner was stoned to death by a mob near Winchester, Illinois, on November 28, 1893.

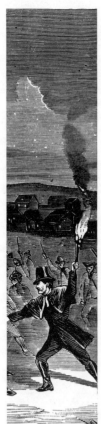

Unruly crowds have been part of "civilization" for as long as people have been gathering together in groups. When frustration, political unrest, panic, or revenge is commonly shared by people in groups, violence can erupt, and loss of life is common.

In the U.S., riots predate independence, by at least a century. Just about any grievance or social wrong imaginable has led to disorder, destruction of property, and loss of life at some point in our history. There has been an "Anti-Rent Riot," a "Street Preaching Riot," the "Portland, Maine Liquor Riot," a "Hungarian Riot," and in Portland, Maine, a "Whorehouse Riot."

Some of the highlights in U.S. riots:

□ May 16, 1771. In Almanance, North Carolina, a riot of anti-tax protestors leaves twenty-nine dead.

□ October, 1834. In Philadelphia, Pennsylvania, Democrats battle Whigs, leaving one dead.

□ August, 1835. In Baltimore, Maryland, when fraud is discovered to have been involved in a bank failure, citizens attempt to punish those involved, leaving twenty dead in the "Anti-Bank Riot."

□ July 8, 1844. In Philadelphia, Pennsylvania, an anti-Irish riot leaves fifty dead.

□ November 4, 1856. In Baltimore, Maryland, the Democrats battle the Know-Nothing Party, leaving eight dead.

□ October 1, 1909. In Los Angeles, California, during a labor riot, a bomb explodes in the L.A. Times Building, killing twenty people.

□ June 22, 1922. In Herrin, Illinois, union strikers in the coal industry massacre scab workers; thirty-six are killed.

☐ August 11-16, 1965. In Los Angeles, California, rioting in the Watts section of the city signals the beginning of mass urban violence by blacks that is a major element of the unrest of the 1960s; thirty-five people are killed.

☐ July 12-17, 1967. In Newark, New Jersey, thousands are injured in riots in the black section of the city; twenty-six are killed.

☐ July 23-30, 1967. In Detroit, Michigan, the National Guard and Army paratroopers were called out to combat rioting in the city's black ghetto; forty people are killed.

During a soccer game in Uruguay in 1972, fans shot two players to prevent a goal from being scored.

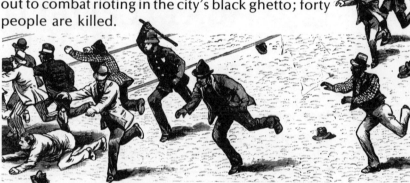

KILLING FEVER

Guiseppe Zangara, age thirty-two, was electrocuted at the state prison in Florida, on March 20, 1933, for the shooting death of Mayor Anton Cermak of Chicago. Zangara shot Cermak and four others in a botched assassination attempt on the life of President-elect Franklin D. Roosevelt on February 15, 1933, in Miami. The assassin claimed that the stomach pains he had suffered for years made him hate presidents and kings. At his trial, he was sentenced to eighty years hard labor for attempted murder — he told the judge, "Don't be stingy, give me 100 years" — and condemned to death for the murder of Chicago's mayor.

At a soccer game in Turkey, forty-one people were killed by gunfire and knifings during a violent dispute among spectators.

*"I have a rendezvous with Death
At some disputed barricade . . .
And I to my pledged word am true,
I shall not fail that rendezvous."*
— Alan Seeger

Chapter Seven

ON THE BATTLEFIELD
Death by
Warfare and Mass Murder

Not content to let the willy-nilly forces of nature control human population, throughout history mankind has contrived to add his mark to the death toll. Seldom since the beginning of recorded history has there been a year unmarked by a war, genocide, or massacre of some kind — men at work, killing other men.

Until recently, however, the destructive tendencies of humans — usually rationalized by political or religious convictions — never rivaled the often calamitous capabilities of nature. Even with the combined total of military and civilian deaths in the worst wars in history, nature was still more effective at killing people. Disease and malnutrition were responsible for many more deaths than the instruments of war — until the twentieth century.

With the invention and use of modern technological weapons, man has been able to mimic the character of nature at its wrathful best. And with the development of nuclear weapons, man has finally outdone nature for the distinction of being the most thorough exterminator.

WAR IS SICK

During the Crimean War, the British Army lost ten times more troops to dysentery than to battle wounds.

"Since argument is not recognized as a means of arriving at truth, adherents of rival dogmas have no method except war by means of which to reach a decision. And war, in our scientific age, means, sooner or later, universal death."
— Bertrand Russell

Of the total fatalities suffered by the military forces of the North and the South in the American Civil War, about 60 percent were caused by disease.

There is probably no finer breeding ground for infectious diseases than an army. Throughout history, the crowded conditions under which soldiers have lived have provided an ideal environment for the rapid spread of deadly germs. Indeed, until relatively recent times, disease was the number one cause of death among all armed forces, including those in European countries and the United States. Not until World War I did combat exceed sickness as the number one killer of American soldiers.

During World War II, the U.S. military had 15,799 fatalities from disease.

Sanitary conditions do not guarantee immunity from disease when large numbers of strangers are suddenly assembled in shared living quarters. Although individuals gradually acquire some immunity from normal exposure in small groups and families, when exposed to strangers bearing new collections of germs and microbes, even a healthy person is likely to experience some new illnesses.

The introduction of an influenza virus, typhoid, tuberculosis, or dysentery to an assembled army often produced widespread fatalities. The first example of this problem in America occurred at Valley Forge during the Revolutionary War. Within a few months, an estimated 3,000 colonial soldiers perished from the combined effects of disease, malnutrition, and hypothermia.

During World War I, 230 American soldiers died from appendicitis.

Florence Nightingale's work was probably the greatest single factor in reducing disease-related deaths of the military. The first major project of her nursing career was a political appointment to the Crimea as a medical aide to the British military. When she arrived in 1854, the army hospital had a mortality rate of 42.7 percent. Six months later, after instituting drastic improvements in sanitation and nursing care, the mortality rate plunged to 2.2 percent.

The wartime fatalities of the French armies during the Napoleanic era caused the average height of Frenchmen to decrease by two-and-a-half inches in fifty years, according to a reference book from 1857.

Nightingale kept detailed records and developed statistical studies which eventually convinced the military that something was drastically wrong with their health care. Her comparison of army life to civilian life showed that, while the average Englishman had a mortality rate of one in a thousand from all causes, the average British soldier suffered from a mortality rate of twenty-three in a thousand, not including deaths on the battlefield.

Nightingale's statistics showed that while at war in the Crimea, the British army suffered such heavy losses that it would have been eradicated without replacements for the dead. In 1855, she demonstrated that the annual mortality rate of the army was 1,174 deaths per thousand, not including those killed in battle. A unit of 100 men, including the replacements brought in during a year just for that unit, would lose an average of 117 men in twelve months.

Her arguments, reforms, and improvements in the Crimea resulted in a troop mortality rate one-third less than that of the noncombat troops "safely" at home in England. Later, in a similar campaign with the British army in India, she helped reduce the mortality rate over a ten-year period from 69 deaths per 1,000 to 18 per 1,000.

In one comparison of the theoretical lethality of weapons, the longbow was found to be as deadly as the early nineteenth century rifle.

_____BODY COSTS

"War is a series of catastrophes which result in victory."
— Georges Clemenceau

Based on the value of the dollar in 1982, these figures represent the cost, per American soldier, of war fatalities:

	Total Cost	Total Fatalities	Cost per Death
Revolutionary War	$120 million	25,324	$ 4,734
War of 1812	87 million	2,260	38,495
Mexican War	82 million	13,283	6,173
Civil War, North	2.3 billion	364,511	6,310
Civil War, South	1 billion	133,821	7,473
Spanish-American War	270 million	2,446	110,384
World War I	32 billion	116,708	274,188
World War II	360 billion	407,316	883,834
Korean War	50 billion	54,246	921,727
Vietnam War	141 billion	57,702	2,436,657

(Total fatalities include non-combatant deaths.)

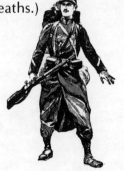

BODY COUNTS

COMBAT FATALITIES

	Total	Army	Navy	Marine	Air Force	Coast Guard
Revolutionary War	4,435	4,044	342	49		
War of 1812	2,260	1,950	265	45		
Mexican War	1,733	1,721	1	11		
Civil War, North	140,414	138,154	2,112	148		
Civil War, South	74,524	N/A	N/A	N/A		
Spanish-American	385	369	10	6		
World War I	53,402	50,510	431	2,461	*	111
World War II	291,557	234,874	36,950	19,733	*	574
Korean War	33,629	27,704	458	4,267	1,200	
Vietnam War	47,253	30,867	1,605	13,066	1,715	

(* Air Corps deaths included with Army.)

NON-COMBAT FATALITIES

(Includes transportation accidents, friendly fire, disease, imprisonment, and missing.)

	Total	Army	Navy	Marine	Air Force	Coast Guard
Revolutionary War	18,500	N/A	N/A	N/A		
War of 1812	N/A					
Mexican War	11,550	11,550				
Civil War, North	224,097	221,374	2,411	312		
Civil War, South	59,297	N/A	N/A			
Spanish-American	2,061	2,061				
World War I	63,195	55,868	6,856	390		81
World War II	115,185	83,400	25,664	4,778		1,343
Korean War	20,617	9,429	4,043	1,261	5,884	
Vietnam War	10,449	7,252	11	1,683	603	

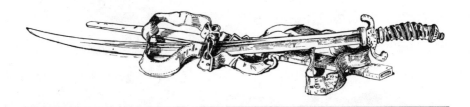

U.S. WAR DEATHS

	U.S. Fatalities	Death Ratio
Revolutionary War	25,324	1 of every 8
War of 1812	2,260	1 of every 127
Mexican War	13,283	1 of every 6
Indian Wars	1,000	1 of every 106
Civil War, North	364,511	1 of every 6
Civil War, South	133,821	1 of every 7
Spanish-American War	2,446	1 of every 125
World War I	116,708	1 of every 40
World War II	407,316	1 of every 40
Korean War	54,246	1 of every 106
Vietnam War	57,702	1 of every 151

The hand grenade is one of the least deadly weapons in modern warfare, accounting for injuries in about 50 percent of the people within twenty feet of its explosion, with less than 10 percent of the injuries being fatal.

The Vietnam War offered soldiers the best chance for survival. But for soldiers fighting for the Union cause during the Civil War, the survival rates were just the opposite — they were the worst in American military history.

MILITARY SERVICE DEATH RATE

Army: 1 out of every 29 soldiers has died.
Navy: 1 out of every 97 has died.
Marines: 1 out of every 26 has died.
Air Force: 1 out of every 321 has died.

Several hundred bomb disposal experts have been killed in European countries since the end of WWII during the removal of leftover munitions from that war. Hundreds of tons of explosives, bombs, and bullets are still scattered across Europe, and the cleanup may take many more years.

These figures indicate only the overall ratio of deaths (both combat and non-combat) in the different branches of the military. No figures were used from pre-Civil War actions because separate totals are not available for all the branches before that time. Also, only the Northern forces were included for the Civil War.

HIGH-POWER FIREPOWER

"When a man hath no freedom to fight
for at home,
Let him combat for that of his neighbors;
Let him think of the glories of Greece and of Rome,
And get knocked on his head for his
labours."
— Lord Byron

In the days before mechanized warfare, the winning army generally averaged about 15 percent casualties; the loser, 20 percent. Back in the 1600s, winning armies suffered as much as 20 percent casualties; the vanquished, 30 percent. As late as World War I, traditional army tactics exposed large numbers of soldiers to concentrated enemy fire and, because most troops were used in direct combat, fatality rates were often as high as 25 percent.

The shift to mechanized warfare at the onset of World War II brought a drastic change in the use of armed forces personnel. With few exceptions, armies had as many as five to ten noncombat personnel supporting each combat soldier. Most casualties occurred in combat, so the overall casualty rate dropped dramatically: the Allied forces averaged about 2 percent casualties, and the Axis forces, about 4 percent in that war.

However, as these casualty rates declined, the amount of ammunition expended grew tremendously. Again, this was a result of changing tactics on the battlefield. With a newly developed dependence on mechanized weapons and transportation, fewer soldiers were in any one area, and more shots had to be fired to increase the possibility of hitting the enemy. One of the interesting lessons of war is that marksmanship is less important than overall volume of fire. This led to the development of artillery and explosive shells to be used against infantry. Even massed rifle fire at close range often resulted in less than half of the targets being hit.

By World War II, the dispersion of soldiers on the battlefield and the use of rapid-fire weapons resulted in 2,425 pounds of ammunition being expended per enemy fatality. Further refinements of weapons, along with even greater dispersion on the battlefield, resulted in 12,346 pounds of ammunition per enemy fatality in the Korean War.

Then came Vietnam, and the age of the big-dollar war was formally introduced. In that conflict, the U.S. shot, dropped, and exploded 39,242 pounds (19.62 tons) of ammunition for each Vietcong fatality. The use of B-52 bombers proved to be the most expensive. On an average high-altitude sortie, these bombers dropped 25 tons of bombs per plane. The results: between 0.7 and 3.4 enemy fatalities.

Still, the B-52 in Vietnam was not the first example of this type of ineffective aerial weapon (ineffective, that is, in producing enemy fatalities). During World War II, the German Armed Forces expected to defeat Great Britain with two newly-developed weapons: the V-1 flying bomb and the V-2 flying rocket. More than 9,200 of the V-1 type were launched toward

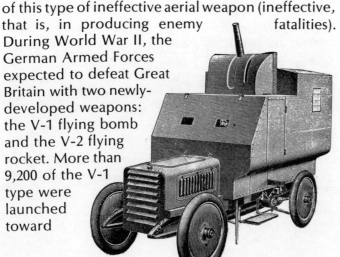

The first deaths from aerial combat were on October 5, 1914 — two German aviators were killed when their biplane was shot down by a French plane.

During World War I, officers in the infantry suffered the highest death rate in the U.S. military — 80.5 fatalities per thousand men. The death rate for enlisted men was 51.7 fatalities per thousand men.

For U.S. military personnel in World War II, there was an overall fatality rate of 20 percent from combat injuries.

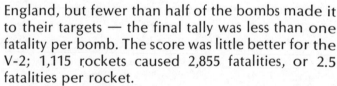

The most destructive air raid in history was on March 9, 1945, before the atomic bomb was dropped on Hiroshima. The U.S. Army Air Corps destroyed more than sixteen square miles of Tokyo in a nighttime bomb attack, using 2,000 tons of bombs dropped from 334 B-29 bombers that shattered and burned 250,000 buildings. The official death count on the ground was 83,793 fatalities, with an unofficial estimate of more than 100,000.

England, but fewer than half of the bombs made it to their targets — the final tally was less than one fatality per bomb. The score was little better for the V-2; 1,115 rockets caused 2,855 fatalities, or 2.5 fatalities per rocket.

Other bombing statistics point out additional problems. For example, one out of every five bombs didn't explode, and many bombs missed their intended targets and caused little damage. A final assessment of World War II bombings showed that it required three tons of bombs to cause one German fatality, and 1.5 tons for a Japanese fatality.

In an attempt to thwart destruction from the air, defenders usually tried to shoot down the offending airplanes. However, the problems involved with anti-aircraft weapons paralleled those with other modern weapons. That is, in order to make a hit, there had to be a lot of firing. In World War II, the Germans fired 12,000 anti-aircraft shells for every Allied plane that was destroyed.

In more modern warfare, various kinds of rockets are used to achieve the same result, but the difficulty remains. In both the Vietnam War and the Arab-Israeli wars, where rockets and missiles were widely used, more than fifty surface-to-air missiles had to be fired for each plane that was brought down. In the 1973 Israeli War, the Arab forces demonstrated another problem with these weapons: they fired 2,100 missiles, which brought down forty Israeli planes — and forty-five of their own.

Some of the big munition expenditures from history:

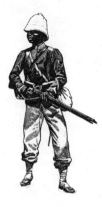

☐ **Crimean War**: The English fired 15 million shots and the Russians lost 21,000 soldiers. The result: 714 shots per fatality. The French fired 29 million shots and killed 51,000 Russians. The result: 569 shots per fatality. The Russians fired 45 million shots, killing

48,000 of the Allied forces. The result: 937 shots per fatality.

☐ **Franco-German War of 1870**: The Germans fired 30 million musket shots and 363,000 artillery shells. The French lost 77,000 soldiers. The result: 394 rounds per fatality.

☐ **World War II**: 2,425 pounds of ammunition (including small arms, artillery, and bombs) were expended for each fatality (U.S.).

☐ **Korean War**: 12,346 pounds of ammunition were expended for each fatality (U.S.).

☐ **Vietnam War**: 39,242 pounds of ammunition were expended for each fatality (U.S.)

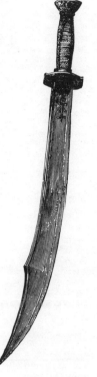

—————————OOPS!
A Short Look At
Some Wartime Accidents

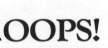

"Many people would sooner die than think. In fact, they do."
— Bertrand Russell

Despite the best of intentions, men at war make as many mistakes as people in other lines of work. Unfortunately, the circumstances and environment of war can easily compound the effects of an accident or miscalculation, resulting in large losses of life.

Some notable American blunders from World War II include:

☐ The USS *Shark*, a submarine, torpedoed and sank the *Arisan Maru* on October 24, 1944. It was a Japanese ship carrying Allied prisoners of war; 1,785 POWs were killed.

At the battle of Solferino in 1859, the Austrian army lost 22,500 soldiers, and the French, 17,200 — in a single day.

During World War I, the Germans sent 103 air strikes against England. From 1914 to 1918, the total loss of life from these raids was 1,413 people.

On March 27, 1945, the last German V-2 rocket hit England, landing in Orpington, Kent at 4:54 pm and killing one person. On March 29, 1945, the last German V-1 flying bomb was launched against England, and was destroyed in the air over Sittingbourne, Kent. A total of 9,200 V-1s were launched toward England, but more than half malfunctioned or were destroyed before hitting a target. Total deaths from the bombs was 6,139, giving the bombs a final score of 1.5 deaths per unit.

☐ The USS *Sealion*, a submarine, torpedoed and sank the *Enoura Maru* on September 12, 1944. It was a Japanese POW transport ship; more than 1,000 POWs from Australia and Great Britain were killed.

☐ Allied planes sank the *Oryoku Maru* on December 15, 1944; more than 900 POWs were killed.

☐ The USS *Barb*, a submarine, torpedoed and sank the *Shinyo Maru* on September 7, 1944; at least 668 POWs were killed.

☐ George Preddy, a U.S. Army Air Force ace in World War II, shot down twenty-six German planes before he was accidentally killed by American anti-aircraft flak.

☐ Schaffhausen, a town in neutral Switzerland, was accidentally bombed by U.S. aircraft on April 1, 1944; fifty people were killed in the attack, for which the town was compensated $3.2 million in damages by the U.S.

☐ The USS *Tang*, a submarine, was sunk by its own torpedo on October 24, 1944, after sinking twenty-four Japanese ships in less than a year. Most of the crew died in the accident. Another U.S. submarine, the USS *Tullibee*, was thought to have been sunk by its own torpedo on March 30, 1944, with only one survivor.

☐ During World War II, the USS *Extractor*, a Navy salvage ship, was accidentally torpedoed and sunk by the USS *Guardfish*, a submarine; six men were killed. This was the only incident of its type in that war for the U.S.

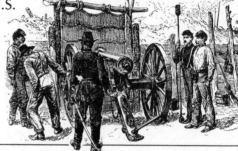

THE BIG LOSERS

"True civilization knows the price of human life but makes the imperishable life of man its transcendent supreme value. It does not fear death, it confronts death, it accepts risk, it requires self-sacrifice — but for aims that are worthy of human life, for justice, for truth, for brotherly love."
— Jacques Maritain

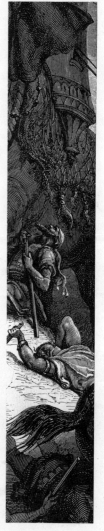

The all-time largest wars in numbers of participants were the two World Wars of this century. Because the size of armies usually influences the number of casualties, these two wars also produced more fatalities than other major wars in history. These countries suffered most:

WORLD WAR I

Germany	1,773,700 military deaths
Russia	1,700,000 military deaths
France	1,357,800 military deaths
Austria-Hungary	1,200,000 military deaths
British Empire	908,371 military deaths
Italy	650,000 military deaths
Romania	335,706 military deaths
Turkey	325,000 military deaths

(The U.S. finished out of the running with "only" 116,708 fatalities.)

WORLD WAR II

U.S.S.R	6,750,000 military deaths
Germany	3,250,000 military deaths
China	1,310,000 military deaths
Japan	1,862,000 military deaths
Poland	664,000 military deaths
United States	407,000 military deaths
Great Britain	357,000 military deaths

Total military deaths in World War I: 8,545,800
Total military deaths in World War II: 15,843,000

GAS PAINS

"Every nation prepares, through its government, to equip itself with the power to hurl death upon its fellow-nations. No people seeks that power; it is governments that seek it."
— Harold J. Laski

The only deaths within the U.S. from enemy action during World War II were on May 5, 1945. A hydrogen balloon launched in Japan and carrying explosives landed in a wooded area of Oregon, where it was discovered and accidentally set off — killing five children and the local minister's wife. The balloon was one of about 1,000 thought to have reached the U.S.

On March 9, 1916, Pancho Villa and 1,500 Mexican guerrillas attacked Columbus, New Mexico, and killed seventeen American citizens.

One of the most sinister developments of World War I was the use of poisonous gases as weapons. After they were first manufactured and deployed in 1915 by the German army, gas warfare gained rapid popularity by all military forces engaged in combat in this conflict. Chlorine was the first to cloud the battlefield, soon followed by phosgene and mustard gas. These were but three of the many gases used during World War I. By war's end, gases accounted for about 20 percent of all munitions used.

The effect of gas differed from other weapons since rather than kill, they usually incapacitated victims of an attack. Gas casualties required a long period of recuperation and therefore extra medical personnel to provide treatment. So, this weapon probably had a bigger impact on warfare than other weapons in use at the time.

The total number of World War I fatalities from gassing is an estimated 91,000. The Russians incurred more injuries and deaths than any other warring nations, primarily because they were least prepared for defense against gas attacks. Other nations quickly developed gas masks which protected their soldiers from the poisons, or at least lessened the effects. The British list a total of 6,062 fatalities from gas; of this number about 10 percent resulted from exposure to misdirected gas attacks by their own side.

An acknowledged problem in estimating the

mortalities caused by gas is its delayed effects. Various chronic health problems from gas eventually caused deaths many years after the exposure. At least one such death reported in England as late as 1981 was attributed to exposure to gas during the first World War. Other problems in accounting for the effects of gas warfare include the lack of records kept for the victims of gas attacks in 1915, the large number of soldiers simply listed as missing, and inadequate information on the cause of death for many prisoners of war.

Warfare results in fatalities of 43 percent for those wounded in the head by artillery fragments; 25 percent for chest wounds; 17 percent for abdominal wounds; and 5 percent from arm wounds.

By the end of the war, all of the major powers had large stockpiles of gas weapons and the facilities to produce even more. Researchers in the U.S., Great Britain, Russia, Germany, and Japan, continued to study new types of gas and other poisons, including germ weapons. Meanwhile, chemical weapons continued to be employed in conflicts around the world, including the Russian Revolution. The French and Spanish also used gas in Morocco; the British in Afghanistan, the Japanese in China, and the Italians in Abyssinia. But due to almost universal negative reactions to the use of gas as a weapon of war, little information could ever be confirmed for the total number of gas-related injuries and fatalities.

Despite public opinion and at least one international treaty outlawing gases, the major powers prepared to use poison gas in World War II. The Germans secretly developed two types of nerve gas, named tabun and sarin, both much more deadly than any of the gases sprayed during World War I. They estimated that either one of the new gases could cause up to 50 percent fatalities on a battlefield.

Throughout the war, the Germans manufactured large quantities of gases, and had stockpiled at least

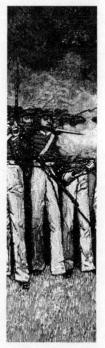

Myrtle, a pet chicken that was parachuted into action in World War II, was killed during the battle of Arnheim in 1944.

Montana State College lost its entire football team in separate actions in World War II. The eleven men who were on the 1940-41 team were the only complete line-up from a U.S. college to be lost in a single war.

70,000 tons of tabun by the end of the war. In addition, they possessed large quantities of mustard gas and phosgene gas, including 500,000 gas bombs to be dropped from planes. Flying bombs and rockets, used with conventional explosives, were also designed to carry nerve gas. The Germans never used any of this gas in World War II — the evidence suggests that they feared the ability of Allied forces to retaliate with their own gases. Some theorize that because Hitler was the victim of a gas attack in World War I, he was adverse to giving his enemies the excuse to gas him again.

Before and during World War II, the British developed, manufactured, and stockpiled a new weapon of their own — anthrax. At one point, they planned to disperse mass quantities of this deadly and highly contagious biological weapon over Berlin. Anthrax is not only deadly (up to an 80 percent mortality rate), it is also capable of reproducing rapidly and it remains toxic for long periods of time. One estimate stated that had Berlin been dosed as planned, the city would still be contaminated today.

Although they were not used for combat in World War II, there were fatalities from poison gases, resulting from mishandling or accidental exposure. The Germans reported at least ten workers who died from accidents at their tabun plant. Hundreds, if not thousands, may have died during testing of chemicals on human subjects. Fatalities from the testing of these weapons have been difficult to prove because of secrecy surrounding their research and use. The Japanese, who tested chemical and biological weapons on human subjects, killed many prisoners of war, mainly Chinese. Evidence from the remains of some of these human guinea pigs show that the Japanese were testing anthrax, cholera, typhoid, the plague, tetanus, and other gases.

The greatest number of fatalities from gas weapons during World War II resulted from an American shipment of mustard gas. The gas was being shipped secretly to Europe to prepare for possible combat use. It was shipped under false papers on merchant ships, and very few people on the ships or in the military were aware of its existence. On December 2, 1943, one of these ships was in the harbor at Bari, Italy, waiting to be unloaded, when a surprise German air raid devastated the harbor area.

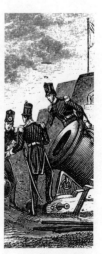

Seventeen ships were sunk, including the one carrying 100 tons of mustard gas. The chemical escaped from the wreck in liquid form along with large clouds of gas. Many sailors were thrown into the water and exposed to the toxic chemical, causing at least seventy deaths. In addition, hundreds of residents of Bari who were exposed to the gas, died. The accident forced the U.S. to admit it had been stockpiling mustard gas; thereafter, it changed its shipping procedures to avoid further accidents.

The first deaths from gas warfare — used by the Germans on Europe's Western Front — were recorded on April 22, 1915.

At the end of World War II, the combined stores of chemical weapons for all the military forces involved totaled at least 500,000 tons, 500 percent more than the total amount of chemical weapons expended in World War I. Despite the atrocities and destruction of the second World War, there was no recorded use of these weapons, despite their deliberate overstocking. However, most military analysts believe that the next time there is a general free-for-all, restraint will evaporate and we will once again experience the gruesome capabilities of chemical armament.

In the American Civil War, 75 percent of all battle casualties were from rifle bullets, and 11 percent were from musket balls.

CENTURIES OF WAR DEATHS

"A single death is a tragedy, a million deaths is a statistic."
— Joseph Stalin

The first civilian death from an air raid in World War II was on March 16, 1940. The Germans attacked the Orkney Islands in Great Britain, and killed one person.

Zulu warriors, using only spears as weapons, killed 1,745 British troops in the battle of Isandhlwana in southeast Africa on January 22, 1879.

The history of war has left the world with a seemingly endless stream of dead bodies. The following are the estimated battle deaths for each century. Civilian fatalities are not included.

	Fatalities
B.C. to 1 A.D.	1,500,000
1 A.D. to 100	1,150,000
101 to 200	75,000
201 to 300	150,000
301 to 400	270,000
401 to 500	230,000
501 to 600	140,000
601 to 700	180,000
701 to 800	400,000
801 to 900	35,000
901 to 1000	9,000
1001 to 1100	161,000
1101 to 1200	75,000
1201 to 1300	475,000
1301 to 1400	245,000
1401 to 1500	125,000
1501 to 1600	630,000
1601 to 1700	1,270,000
1701 to 1800	2,106,000
1801 to 1900	4,100,000
1900 to present	31,106,000

Total to date: 45,000,000

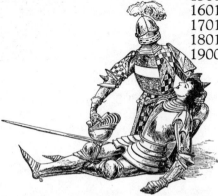

CIVILIAN WAR DEATHS

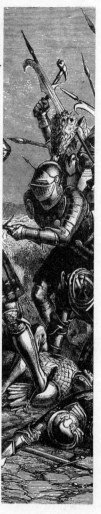

"It is necessary that our civilization build its temple on mountains of corpses, on an ocean of tears and on the death cries of men without number."
— Count Gottlieb Von Haeseler

With the advance of warfare technology, more and more civilians have become involved in the destruction of war. Historically, battles matched armies against one another in fixed engagements. However, with the development of war machines, particularly the airplane, there was no longer any guarantee that the intended victims would be enemy soldiers. Civilian deaths escalated rapidly throughout World War I, preparing the world for future wars, when anyone was fair game.

The civilian population of Europe accounted for about 5 percent of the casualties in World War I. This figure grew to 50 percent in World War II. The latter figure included almost 20 percent of the entire population of Poland, and at least 10 percent of the populations of both Russia and Germany. Some of the largest concentrations of civilian fatalities were due to airplane bombings. In four successive air raids over Hamburg, Germany, the British dropped 8,261 tons of bombs, almost destroying the city and killing at least 60,000 people.

The U.S. eclipsed this feat on the night of March 9, 1945, when 2,000 tons of bombs were dropped on Tokyo, causing the most destruction from any air raid in history, including the atomic bombs dropped on Hiroshima and Nagasaki. The Tokyo air raids burned more than sixteen square miles of the city, destroyed over a quarter-million buildings, and killed close to 100,000 people.

THE
ULTIMATE WEAPON

On April 26, 1937, the German Air Force, at the invitation of Francisco Franco, experimented with aerial saturation bombing on the city of Guernica, Spain, at noon on market day; at least 1,654 people (24 percent of the population) were killed.

"Hitherto man had to live with the idea of death as an individual; from now onward mankind will have to live with the idea of its death as a species."
— Arthur Koestler

On August 6, 1945, the world's second atomic bomb was dropped on Hiroshima (the first bomb was detonated as a test near Alamogordo, New Mexico, on July 16, 1945) and the world's third atomic bomb was dropped on Nagasaki on August 9 of the same year. No one questions that both of the bombs used against the Japanese caused immense physical damage and loss of life. However, there is no accurate figure for the total deaths from these explosions. This is because large numbers of undocumented Japanese military personnel and civilians were either passing through the two cities at the time of detonation, or were unofficially living there. And, in many cases, the power of the bomb left no traces of human tissue to contribute to the body count. The unknown and poorly documented cases of radiation poisoning added further confusion.

The following are just some of the available estimates of deaths:

	Hiroshima
Governor's report, Hiroshima Prefecture, August 20, 1945	32,959
Public Health Section report, Hiroshima, August 25, 1945	46,185
Police Department report, Hiroshima, November 30, 1945	78,150
Official Report of City of Hiroshima, March 8, 1946	47,185
Survey Section report, Hiroshima, August 10, 1946	118,661
United States-Japan Joint Survey report, 1951	64,602
U.S. Strategic Bombing Survey	70,000- 80,000
Japanese Council Against A- and H-Bombs, 1961	119,000- 133,000

— (Does not include 32,900 estimated military personnel)

	Nagasaki
Prefecture report, Nagasaki, August 31, 1945	19,748
Prefecture report, Nagasaki, October 23, 1945	23,753
Private estimate, Japan, January, 1946	29,398-37,507
Report, Great Britain, c.1947	39,500
A-Bomb Records Preservation Committee, Nagasaki, 1949	73,884
United States-Japanese Joint Survey Report, 1951	29,570-39,214
United States-Japanese Joint Survey Report, 1956	39,000
U.S. Strategic Bombing Survey	40,000

——————A-BOMBS KILL AMERICANS

"Death must take me for someone else."
— Samuel Beckett

Although it is not an official secret, few people know that there were Allied Prisoners of War in both Hiroshima and Nagasaki when the atomic bombs were detonated in 1945. American servicemen were listed among the soldiers in both places.

Nagasaki had two POW camps. The closest one was about a mile from the center of the explosion; the other was more than six miles away from the center. British, Dutch, Australian, and American troops were interned in these camps, and, although exact numbers are not known, it is believed these troops totaled about 2,000 prisoners. Investigations conducted by Allied sources after the Japanese surrender failed to provide conclusive casualty figures. However, other sources, including a Japanese report, indicate a total of sixty to eighty POW deaths could be attributed to the bomb.

No POW camps in Hiroshima were directly affected by the bomb that exploded over that city. However, several groups of American flyers,

Out of 2,500 German generals in WWII, 786 were killed in the war: 41 percent died of unspecified causes; 32 percent were killed in battle; 10 percent committed suicide; 6 percent died from wounds; 5 percent were executed by the Allies; and 3 percent were executed by order of Hitler.

The total battle deaths on all sides during World War I was greater than all of the deaths from all of the wars for the preceding 100 years.

During a mass parachute drop at Fort Bragg, North Carolina, on November 17, 1953, a C-119 crashed, killing fifteen men. Nine of them were paratroopers who were hit by the falling plane on its way down.

Three U.S. destroyers sank in a typhoon near the Philippines, taking 730 men with them, on December 17, 1944. This was the worst storm disaster in U.S. Navy history.

captured after they had abandoned their aircraft on previous missions, were being held by the Hiroshima police in that city. Most of these Americans died in the blast, or shortly thereafter. Japanese records show that twenty Americans were killed by the bomb. But because names and serial numbers are not listed for every case, the Japanese only accept ten American deaths as conclusive. At least a few of these deaths were due to stoning by Japanese civilians after the bomb had exploded.

Official U.S. records list only one American fatality in Hiroshima; the cause of death being listed as "atomic explosion." The Pentagon does not deny that more American servicemen might have been in Hiroshima and killed by the blast, but their policy is not to list deaths as official unless undeniable proof exists — thereby eliminating other possible causes of death. A conclusive report will probably never be possible as little evidence survived either the Hiroshima blast or the accidental destruction of U.S. military records in a fire in St. Louis in 1973.

CHEESE WAR

Two sailors on board a Brazilian warship in the mid-1800s were killed by pieces of cheese that had been fired from a Uruguayan ship during a naval battle. When the Uruguayan ship ran out of regular ammunition for its cannon, the captain had ordered them loaded with Dutch cheeses. One of the cheeses hit the mast on the Brazilian ship and shattered, killing the sailors and causing the Brazilian warship to retreat from the field of fire.

DEADLY PERSECUTIONS

"The history of the world which is still taught to our children is essentially a series of race murders."
— Sigmund Freud

Select any point in history and, no doubt, some group has suffered persecution at the hands of another group. Persecuted groups have undergone torment because of religious or political beliefs. At the least, they have endured humiliation, physical abuse, and general societal mistreatment; at the worst, death to individuals or genocide.

The Nazis' incredible efficiency and ruthless determination marked their attempted genocide of the Jews as the biggest example of group persecution. However, they were not the first to indulge in this behavior against Jews, as this brief history of Jewish persecution suggests.

☐ **1096**: 10,000 killed during the first Crusade in France.

☐ **1096**: 5,000 killed during the first Crusade in Germany, including 1,100 at Mainz.

☐ **1236**: 2,500 killed during the third Crusade in France.

☐ **1298-1299**: 3,500 killed in the Rindfleisch Massacre in Germany.

☐ **1320**: 700 killed in the Shepard's Movement in southern France.

☐ **1391-1492**: 100,000 killed in Spain.

☐ **1336-1337**: 6,000 killed in the Armieder Massacres in Germany.

☐ **1348-1350**: 15,000 killed in Germany, victims of ignorance and fear of the Black Plague, including 6,000 burned at Mainz.

Alfred Chenfalls — a man who volunteered to be a live decoy for Winston Churchill in World War II — was killed in June, 1943, when the plane he was on was shot down by the Germans over the Bay of Biscay. The British knew that the Germans would try to shoot the plane down, but did not alter its flight plan in order to preserve their big secret — the ability to translate the German secret code. Actor Leslie Howard was on the same plane, and was also killed.

☐ **1490**: 70,000 killed in Spain.

☐ **1648**: 80,000 killed in the Ukraine in Russia during a revolt against Polish rule.

☐ **1881**: Several hundred killed in Russia.

☐ **1903-1906**: 800 killed in Russia by a right-wing group called the "Black Hundreds."

☐ **1917-21**: 6,000 killed by the Ukrainian National Army.

☐ **1917-1921**: 6,000 killed by the Ukrainian National Army.

☐ **1917-1921**: 60,000 killed by the White Armies in Russia during the revolution.

☐ **1930-1945**: 6 million killed by Nazis in a planned

And, of course, the Jews have not been alone in the bloody history of genocide on the planet. Some of the other significant persecutions include:

☐ **1500 to 1700**: 15,000,000 native South Americans killed during colonization.

☐ **1492 to late 1800s**: 600,000 American Indians killed during colonization.

☐ **1770 to 1900**: 245,000 Australian aborigines killed during colonization.

☐ **1800 to 1950s**: 21,000,000 Africans killed in the Congo during European exploitation of the rubber trees.

☐ **mid 1800s**: 1,000,000 Africans killed by the Zulus during expansion of their empire.

☐ **1930s**: 10,000,000 Russians killed during the Stalin Communist purges.

☐ **1894 to 1915**: 1,500,000 Armenians killed by Turks.

The total battle deaths on all sides during World War I was greater than all of the deaths from all of the wars for the preceding 100 years.

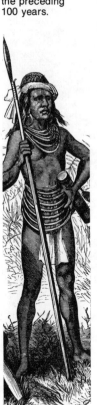

IN THE NAME OF GOD

"Hooded in angry mist, the sun goes down:
Steel-grey the clouds roll out across the sea;
Is this a Kingdom? Then give Death the crown,
For here no emperor hath won, save He."
— Herbert Asquith

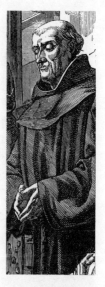

In the history of persecutions and genocides, which continues to this day, the blood has always flowed most freely when one religious group opposes another. Some of the significant rivalries:

☐ **Christian versus Moslem**. The Crusades resulted in thousands of fatalities on both sides.

☐ **Catholic versus Protestant**. The Thirty Years' War in Europe ended in 1648, after more than 3,000,000 fatalities.

☐ **Catholic versus Protestant**. Twenty-four people died in riots between these two religious factions in Philadelphia in 1844. Two Catholic churches were burned.

☐ **Catholic versus Puritan**. In the Battle of the Severn (River) in January, 1655, about twenty people were killed on both sides in Maryland, at the future site of Annapolis.

☐ **Christian versus Heretic**. The Inquisition during the Middle Ages and surrounding periods resulted in the deaths of thousands of non-conforming Christians and Jews in Europe.

☐ **Christian versus Witch**. Pagans got the worst of it during persecution by the Christians from about 1400 to 1700 in Europe, with women most often the victims. More than 1,000,000 died during this purge. At least 133 witches were burned to death in Saxony on one day in 1589, and 1,000 were burned to death in one year in Como, Italy, during the same period.

There were at least several dozen German priests stationed in Hiroshima at the time the atomic bomb was dropped, and several survived the blast.

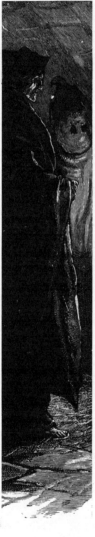

☐ **Christian versus Quaker**. Hundreds of members of the Society of Friends were killed in Europe in the 17th century. In the American colonies, where the Quakers had fled to avoid persecution, four were hanged in 1661 on Boston Commons.

☐ **Christian versus Mormon**. Hundreds of followers of Joseph Smith and his Church of Jesus Christ of Latter-Day Saints were killed in mob violence and murder (including Joseph Smith and his brother) during the 1830s and 1840s.

☐ **Irish Catholic versus Irish Protestant**. 2,380 have been killed in clashes and terrorism in Ireland since the late 1960s. In one famous riot in the U.S., Irish immigrants, split between the two factions, clashed in New York City on July 12, 1871, and fifty-two died.

☐ **Jew versus Arab** (1948 to present). Thousands have been killed in wars and terrorist activity between Israel and the Arab states.

☐ **Hindu versus Moslem**. 500,000 have been killed in violence in India, Bangladesh, and Pakistan.

☐ **Christian versus Moslem**. More than 500,000 died during violent clashes between native groups in northern Sudan, from 1955 through 1972.

☐ **Greek Orthodox Christian versus Turkish Moslem**. In Cyprus, thousands of fatalities in 1974 were the result of traditional animosity between these two groups.

☐ **Moslem versus Bahai**. In Iran, several hundred have been killed in recent years in clashes between the militant state religion and the Bahais.

☐ **Christian versus Sunni (Moslem) versus Shiite (Moslem) versus Druze (Moslem)**. Fighting in Lebanon since 1975 has claimed at least 100,000 lives.

☐ **Sikh versus Hindu**. In India, militant Sikhs agitating for more power and freedom have run up against the Hindu military forces, leaving more than 1,000 dead. Anti-Sikh rioting after the assassination of Indira Gandhi caused the deaths of several thousand more.

☐ **Buddhist versus Hindu**. Sri Lanka, despite its idyllic environment, played host to violence between the Hindu Tamil minority and the Buddhist majority, in which about 400 lives were lost in 1983.

☐ **Shiite versus Sunni** (1980-present). 200,000 have been killed so far in this war between Iran and Iraq.

Dachau, a concentration camp run by the Germans from 1933 to 1945, had more than 206,000 prisoners, of which at least 32,000 were known to have died; about 1,500 of them were catholic priests.

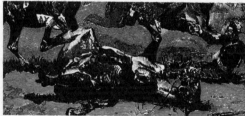

——HORSE MEAT

Soldiers aren't the only ones who get killed in battle. Up until World War I, when horses were still a major part of war, it was common for more horses than men to be killed in a fight. Some of the bad ones for horses were:

September has been the deadliest month this century for fatalities in battle. The second deadliest month is July.

Napoleon's Invasion of Russia, 1812: 185,400 French horses killed.

Battle of Waterloo: 5,572 Allied horses killed.

Crimean War: 3,679 British horses killed.

Battle of Gettysburg, American Civil War: 1,629 horses killed on both sides.

Battle of Chickamauga, American Civil War: 406 horses killed on both sides.

Siege of Plevna, Russian-Turkish War: 22,000 Russian horses killed.

*"The Democracy of Death.
It comes equally to us all, and makes us all
equal when it comes."*
— John Donne

Chapter Eight

NATURE'S WAY
Death from Natural Phenomena

The violence of natural forces has opposed the peace and security of mankind since the beginning of civilization. No man-made device or activity, with the exception of the atom bomb, has been able to rival the deadly efficiency of the powers unleashed by the earth and its atmosphere.

Even with modern planning, regulated building methods, and warning systems, thousands of people die every year from the effects of tornadoes, hurricanes, floods, earthquakes, volcanos, and other "weapons" of nature. In India, thousands of people die every year from floods and cyclones, and as many as 20,000 deaths can be attributed to snake bite. In the U.S., snakes only kill an average of six people per year, but another 100 people are killed by tornadoes.

While these forces of nature do not take as many lives as disease and other human health problems, their overall effect is often greater. The sudden impact of a natural disaster makes front page news, while the fatality rate from malaria often doesn't even appear in the newspaper. The impact of illness on the human body can now be kept to a minimum with improved standards of living, nutrition, and diet. While a reasonable income can shield the middle and upper classes against the ravages of disease and malnutrition, no amount of money can buy protection from the heavy guns of nature's lethal forces. There is no effective protection against the power of a volcano or a flash flood, or the force of hurricane winds or avalanches. The only safe defense against these deadly powers remains the same for rich and poor — flee for your life.

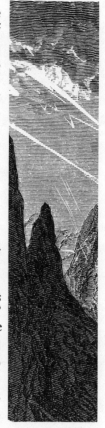

DISASTER FATALITIES

"There are so many ways of us dying it's astonishing any of us choose old age."
— Beryl Bainbridge

The average number of deaths from natural disasters varies from continent to continent. Due to differences in building construction, population density, and advance warning systems, some places are much more deadly than others. These figures were compiled from a twenty-year survey:

	Number of Disasters	Total Fatalities	Average Fatalities per Disaster
North America	210	7,965	37
Central America and Caribbean	49	14,820	302
South America	45	15,670	348
Africa	17	18,105	1,065
Europe (not U.S.S.R.)	85	19,575	230
Asia (not U.S.S.R.)	297	361,410	1,216
Australia	13	4,310	332
TOTAL	716	441,855	618

BOLTS FROM THE BLUE

"The heavens thundered and the air shone with frequent fire; and all things threatened men with instant death."
— Virgil

On the average, lightning kills about one person a year while he or she is talking on a telephone. A similar fate occurs to about one person a year while using a CB radio.

On April 22, 1932, a bolt of lightning in Elgin, Manitoba, hit a flock of wild geese, killing 52 of the birds and providing dinner for many Elgin households.

At a baseball game in Florida on July 31, 1949, a lightning bolt hit the infield, cutting a ditch twenty feet long, and killing the shortstop, first baseman, second baseman, and injuring thirty spectators.

It's not news that lightning can be deadly; hundreds of people are killed each year by lightning. Learning to come indoors for safety during thunderstorms is basic to a child's education. However, the unfortunate truth is that no place — indoors or outdoors — is entirely safe, as evidenced by these incidents:

A single bolt of lightning hit an army arsenal in New Jersey on July 10, 1926. It destroyed every structure within 2,700 feet and killed sixteen people. Debris from the explosion was blown as far away as twenty-two miles. In this case, the secondary effects were more lethal than the lightning itself.

On December 23, 1975, a lightning bolt struck a shed in Rhodesia and killed twenty-one people. This is the largest death toll from a single bolt. The largest lightning kill in U.S. history took place on July 12, 1961, in North Carolina. Eight people, who had taken shelter from the storm in a tobacco barn, were killed by one lightning bolt.

The survival rate for lightning strikes is only 50 percent, making lightning the most fatal force in nature. The final statistics on lightning deaths are not always complete; many more people die from the aftereffects of a lightning strike — explosions, building fires, forest fires, and electrocution from downed power lines — and these figures do not always make it into the lightning toll.

But the destruction of life from lightning is not restricted to humans. Many animals are constantly exposed to the weather, and four-legged animals are connected to the grounding effects of the earth with twice the number of limbs as humans. In an eight-week period during the summer of 1977, lightning killed seventeen calves and twenty-four cows in Alabama, twelve cows in Illinois, eleven in South Carolina, twenty-one in Florida, seven in Idaho, sixteen in Pennsylvania, and ten in Minnesota.

In the case of herd animals such as sheep and cattle, a single bolt can cause multiple deaths; fatalities in herds often number more than ten from a single strike. On July 22, 1918, in the Wasatch National Forest in Utah, a lightning bolt killed 504 sheep, the record in the U.S.

In the 1700s, in one 33-year period, 400 churches were struck by lightning in Europe, and 100 bell-ringers were killed.

A freak windstorm hit the eastern coast of the U.S. between New Jersey and southern New England on the Fourth of July, 1949. With gusts more than sixty miles-per-hour, hundreds of small boats were capsized and nine people drowned.

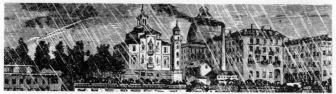

Lightning rods are a relatively efficient means of diminishing the harmful effects of lightning. But at one time, it was believed that bolts were of divine origin and could be warded off only by prayer. Some church bells used to be inscribed with a Latin phrase, "Fulgara Frango," which means "I break up the lightning flashes." Believing that they could indeed dispel the flashes, people rang the bells during thunderstorms. However, not only did this not have the desired effect, but church towers were struck more often than other structures, both because of their height and the metal in the bells. Over a 33-year span in the 1700s, 400 churches were struck and more than 100 bell-ringers were killed.

In this century, Asia has had the heaviest toll of fatalities from natural disasters, and Australia the least.

In 1769, a lightning strike at a church in St. Nazaire, Bresica, set off a cache of gunpowder being stored in the building, and killed 3,000 people. Another strike on a church, also with gunpowder on the premises, caused the deaths of 4,000 people on the Island of Rhodes in 1856.

STRIKE STATS

Only about half of all lightning-caused fatalities take place out-of-doors. The breakdown for outdoor lightning deaths:

- ☐ 38 percent die while taking part in water activities
- ☐ 16 percent die while camping and picnicking
- ☐ 14 percent die while golfing
- ☐ 2 percent die while riding horses (often the rider will be killed without harm to the horse)
- ☐ 21 percent die in miscellaneous accidents
- ☐ 9 percent die at athletic events

Other strike stats:
- ☐ About 75 percent of lightning deaths are male.
- ☐ About 22 percent of lightning victims are under the age of eighteen.
- ☐ About 70 percent of lightning deaths occur in the afternoon.
- ☐ Worst months for lightning deaths: June, July, August.
- ☐ Worst state for lightning deaths (most fatalities): Florida.
- ☐ Worst spot in the U.S. for lightning strikes: Clearwater Forest in Idaho.
- ☐ States with highest fatality rates from

In a report issued in 1847 by Sir William Snow Harris in England, he stated that 220 ships had been hit and 90 sailors killed by lightning in the previous ten years.

On July 17, 1974, a lightning bolt in Oquawka, Illinois, killed a circus elephant while it was chained to a tree.

On September 7, 1970, a lightning bolt hit a group of football players in a huddle during a game in St. Petersburg, Florida. Two players were killed.

lightning strikes: Pennsylvania, Michigan, New York, North Carolina, Ohio, Mississippi, Louisiana, Arkansas, and Oklahoma.

☐ States with lowest fatality rates from lightning attacks: California, Nevada, Washington, North Dakota, and South Dakota.

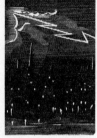

THE HAIL OF IT

"There is a reaper, whose name is Death,
And with his sickle keen,
He reaps the bearded grains at a breath,
And the flowers that grow between."
— Longfellow

Hailstones killed 246 people during a storm in 1888 near New Delhi, India. The same storm killed 1,600 farm animals.

Thunderstorms can mean double trouble. Danger lies not only in lightning bolts, but also in the hail that sometimes accompanies these storms. Hailstones have been known to kill people. These small stones made of ice and snow are produced in cloud formations associated with thunderstorms. They are generally less than a half-inch in diameter and are usually only destructive to farm crops. However, when their size increases, so does the threat to humans.

Six children were killed by hail the size of hens' eggs in a storm in Rumania in 1928.

Weather records from around the world list many fatalities due to hail. On April 30, 1888, near New Delhi, India, 246 people were killed by a storm that produced hailstones described as being as large as cricket balls. At least 1,600 farm animals also died from this aerial bombardment. Another 200 victims of hail died in a storm in the Hunan Province in China on June 19, 1932. On May 1, 1928, in Rumania,

On April 30,
1979, in Fort
Collins,
Colorado, a
small child was
killed by
hailstones
while being
held by its
mother.

six children were killed by hail the size of hens' eggs. A hailstorm in Greece on June 13, 1930, claimed twenty-two lives. Hailstones that weighed up to two pounds killed twenty-three people in Russia in a storm on July 10, 1923.

Animals, too, have suffered from these projectiles from the sky. On July 15, 1978, hail the size of baseballs killed more than 200 sheep in Montana. A large storm in Alberta, Canada, on July 14, 1953, killed 36,000 ducks; another storm a few days later killed 27,000 ducks.

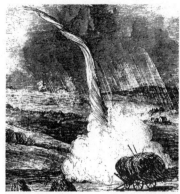

TWISTERS

*"Blessed be death that cuts in marble
What would have sunk in dust."*
— Edna St. Vincent Millay

On the average, about 850 tornadoes a year can be expected in the U.S., and most tornado fatalities will occur in the Southeast. Although tornado season is generally considered April through June and most of these wind funnels show up in midwestern and southern states, tornadoes have occurred in every month of the year and in every state in the U.S.

The great
Siberian
meteor of 1908
only stunned
one native, but
his hut was
destroyed and
many of his
reindeer were
killed.

Some of the big twisters:

		Fatalities
Natchez, Mississippi	May 7, 1840	317
Midwest and South	February 19, 1884	884
Illinois, Indiana, Missouri	March 18, 1925	689
Alabama	March 21, 1932	268
Tupelo, Mississippi	April 5, 1936	216
Gainesville, Georgia	April 6, 1936	203
Midwestern states	April 11, 1965	257
Midwest, East, and South	April 3, 1974	307

From 1970 to 1980 there were a total of 8,573 tornadoes in the U.S., with 986 fatalities. The National Oceanic and Atmospheric Administration has projected that there will be 7,000 tornadoes — with about 1,000 fatalities — in our current decade.

Deadliest month   **April**
Safest month   **July**
Deadliest area   **Southeast**
Deadliest state   **Mississippi**
Deadliest time of day   **Late afternoon**

——BLOW BY BLOW

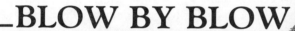

"Death is here and death is there,
Death is busy everywhere,
All around, within, beneath,
Above is death — and we are death."
— Shelley

Some of the notable hurricanes in this century in the U.S.:

		Fatalities
Galveston, Texas	August 27-Sep. 15, 1900	6,000
Southern Florida	Sep. 6-Sep. 20, 1928	1,836
S. New England	Sep. 10-22, 1938	600
Gulf Coast	June 25-28, 1957	390

A devastating hurricane hit Galveston, Texas, in September, 1900, leaving betwen 6,000 and 7,000 dead.

Some of the big blows from other parts of the world:

		Fatalities
India	October, 1737	300,000
India	October, 1876	200,000
India	June, 1882	100,000
East Pakistan	May, 1961	22,000
East Pakistan	May, 1965	36,000

AVALANCHE IN ENGLAND?

"Fear no more the heat of the sun
Nor the furious winter's rages;
Thou thy worldly task has done,
Home art gone and ta'en thy wages."
— Shakespeare

During World War I, in the European Alps, avalanches were deliberately started in order to inflict casualties on the opposing armies. One estimate suggests that more than 50,000 soldiers were killed using this tactic.

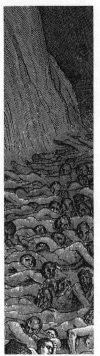

Although England is not known for heavy snowfall or for its mountains, on December 27, 1836, eight people were killed by an avalanche in southern England. In the town of Lewes where a large section of hillside had been removed by workers in order to gain access to quarry stone, an unusual amount of snow fell over a period of days and accumulated in the gash cut into the hill. Residents of the homes adjacent to the site watched as the winds built the snow into an ominous mass. Many felt that there was a threat to their safety and left, but others ignored the danger. Those who stayed died inside seven dwellings that were hit and smashed when the avalanche occurred.

The event is recorded on a stone monument in the courtyard of the local church. The inscription notes: "This tablet is placed by subscription to record an awful instance of the uncertainty of human life . . ."

Although relatively rare, rock avalanches kill more people than any other type of landslide. Such avalanches, induced by earthquakes, usually begin with rock masses falling or sliding from steep, high slopes. Even on gentle slopes, such slides can attain velocities of hundreds of miles per hour.

Precisely such an avalanche caused the death of 18,000 people in Peru in 1970. Only four rock avalanche-related deaths have occurred in North

America during the twentieth century. Several rockslides have been reported in California and Alaska during the past five years, but none have produced fatalities.

Avalanches and landslides have been a common occurrence throughout history. These are some of the notable ones:

The largest death toll from an avalanche in the U.S. is 110, from a snow slide on March 1, 1910, in Wellington, Washington.

			Fatalities
Plurs, Switzerland	September 4, 1618	(snow)	1,500
Wellington, Washington	March 1, 1910	(snow)	110
Italian Alps	December 13, 1916	(snow)	10,000
Northern Assam, India	February 15, 1949	(landslide)	500
Austrian Alps	January 22, 1951	(snow)	222
Blons, Austria	January 12, 1954	(snow)	200
Tokyo, Yokahama, Japan	June, 1961	(landslide)	270
Kiev, U.S.S.R.	March 30, 1961	(landslide)	145
Ranrahirca, Peru	January 10, 1962	(snow)	3,500
Brazil	January 11, 1966	(landslide)	550
Aberfan, Wales	October 21, 1966	(coal slag)	144
Congo	March 8, 1968	(landslide)	154
Peru	1970	(rockslide)	18,000

KILLER FOGS

"I must go in, for the fog is rising."
— Emily Dickinson's dying words
(1886)

A heavy snowstorm in New York City on December 19, 1948, caused the deaths of at least five people. The snow reached a depth of 19.6 inches during the storm.

Fog is as common to England as Yorkshire pudding, but only recently has the lethal properties of certain types of fog become apparent. Before modern controls on pollution — particularly noxious emissions from the burning of coal — the atmospheric conditions that generated fog would also trap poisonous fumes, causing severe health problems for people who lived in the vicinity. In

1953, a particularly heavy fog permeated London for four days — resulting in the deaths of 4,000 people.

A similar type of fog in the Meuse Valley in Europe killed sixty people in 1930. In the steel mill town of Donora, Pennsylvania, nineteen people died from such a fog on Halloween in 1948.

Although there are hundreds of recorded instances of meteorites hitting Earth, there are no known human fatalities resulting from the impact between humans and these rocks from outer space.

———LAVA DEATHS

"Golden lads and girls all must,
As chimney-sweepers, come to dust."
— Shakespeare

The Roman writer, Pliny the Elder, died on August 24, 79 A.D., after approaching Mount Vesuvius during an eruption. He was attempting to study this natural phenomenon and expired after inhaling poisonous fumes from the volcano.

In 1783, a huge lava flow occurred in Iceland. Coursing from a large fissure that was estimated to be more than twenty miles long, the lava flowed in two separate waves, one of which was at least 100 feet high. More than 9,000 people — about 20 percent of Iceland's total population at the time — and most of the cattle on the island were killed. Many people were killed by huge floods of water caused by lava flowing into lakes. Others died from suffocation from volcanic fumes and ash.

VOLCANO		Fatalities
Pompeii	August 24, 79 A.D.	20,000
Mt. Vesuvius, Italy	December 17, 1631	4,000
Mt. Laki, Iceland	June-July, 1783	10,000
Krakatoa, East Indies	August 27, 1883	36,000
Martinique, West Indies	May 8, 1902	40,000
Indonesia	April 25, 1966	1,000

_____EATEN BY THE EARTH

*"I begin to regard the death and mangling
of a couple thousand men as a small
affair, a kind of morning dash — and it
may be well that we become so hardened."*
— William Tecumseh Sherman

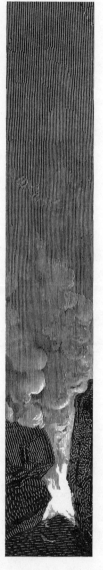

According to Waverly Persons of the National Earthquake Information Center of Golden, Colorado, major earthquakes — registering 7.0-7.9 on the Richter Scale — have occurred at the rate of eighteen per year over the past century. Great earthquakes — registering 8.0 or more — have occurred at the rate of one per year throughout the century.

Significant earthquakes are classified as those registering 6.5 or more on the Richter scale. Below is a table of significant earthquakes worldwide since 1975 and their related death tolls.

	Significant Earthquakes	Fatalities
1975	52	2,372
1976	79	278,252
1977	42	2,819
1978	62	15,194
1979	59	1,571
1980	71	7,134
1981	51	3,724
1982	56	3,335
1983	70	2,270

Some people fear being swallowed by giant cracks in the ground when earthquakes occur. Although most earthquakes do not create fissures large enough to accommodate human bodies, there have been witnessed accounts of people being "devoured" by the planet during violent seismic activity.

In 1692, many people were reported lost in giant cracks and crevices at Port Royal, Jamaica. (Some were later spat out with quantities of water and sand.) Other tremor tales include a story from the Philippines, where a boat was said to have disappeared into one fissure, and a child into another. In one California earthquake, a cow was engulfed in a fissure which then closed, leaving only the tail showing.

Earthquakes do cause great losses of life, mostly from the collapse of buildings. Also, fires started by earthquakes are not easy to put out because water pressure is often decreased by broken water pipes. Since the beginning of the twentieth century, it has been estimated that more than 850,000 people have been killed by earthquakes throughout the world. In the history of the planet, more than 75 million people have died from this natural killer.

Some of the big quakes in history:

Robert E. Lee died in 1870 in Lexington, Virginia, just after a flood had swept through the town. Because the water had carried away all of the available coffins, a search was undertaken to find one in which to bury the General. The only one found had been built for a child; in order to fit him in, he was buried with his boots off.

		Fatalities
Shensi Province, China	January 24, 1556	830,000
Yeddo, Japan	1703	190,000
Calcutta, India	October 11, 1737	300,000
San Francisco, California	April 18, 1906	1,000
Kansu Province, China	December 16, 1920	200,000
Japan	September 1, 1923	140,000
Turkey	December 27, 1939	100,000
Tangshan, China	July 28, 1976	242,000
Bucharest, Rumania	March 4, 1977	1,541
Taba, Iran	September 16, 1978	25,000
Naples, Italy	November 23, 1980	3,000

WASHED AWAY

"Like the dew on the mountain,
Like the foam on the river,
Like the bubble on the fountain,
Thou art gone, and forever!"
— Walter Scott

The most destructive flood in this century was on the Huang He River in China in 1928; almost 4 million people drowned.

The worst floods since 1900 in the U.S.:

		Fatalities
Ohio River and tributaries	March, 1913	467
Texas	December, 1913	177
Arkansas River (Colorado)	June, 1921	120
Texas	September, 1921	215
Mississippi Valley	Spring, 1927	313
Ohio River and lower Mississippi River basins	January-February, 1937	139
New England	September, 1938	600
Northeast states	August, 1955	187
James River (Virginia)	August, 1969	153
Buffalo Creek (West Virginia)	February, 1972	125
Black Hills (South Dakota)	June, 1972	237
Thompson Canyon (Colorado)	July, 1976	139

(Where states are listed, more than one river flooded.)

MOON KILLS

"Pale Death, with impartial step, knocks
at the poor man's cottage and the palaces
of kings."
— Horace

A cyclone in India in 1737 killed over 300,000 people; another 300,000 died in a cyclone in Bangladesh in 1970.

Moonstruck may indeed be more than just a romantic inclination; it could describe an actual physical condition. For years, popular belief has held that the moon — especially when it is full — affects some people in strange ways. Recently, this notion has piqued the interest of a few members of

More than 75 million people are estimated to have been killed by earthquakes in the history of the planet.

On January 10, 1951, a carpenter on the roof of his house in Dusseldorf, Germany, was killed by a six-foot-long piece of ice that speared his body.

the scientific community, thereby picking up a semblance of validity. Various forms of deviant activity, including murder, suicide, assault, insanity, and juvenile delinquency have all been linked to phases of the moon, and most commonly, to the period when the moon is full.

A few theories have been advanced to explain this phenomenon. Some state that it involves the gravitational forces at work on the brain. Others contend that deviant behavior is the result of alterations in the body's basic rhythmic cycles caused by the increased amount of light at night. Whatever the reasons, there are some interesting statistics to be considered:

□ During one full moon period in Iran about 1980, more than 100 young Iranians attempted suicide.
□ The My Lai massacre in Vietnam occurred during a full moon in 1969.
□ In a study of the murder rate in Dade County, Florida, over a fifteen-year period, the highest number of murders occurred during full moons.
□ Studies of suicides in Buffalo, New York, show a distinct correlation with the periods of full moon.

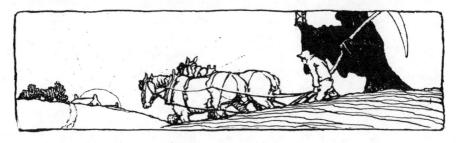

□ The world's largest sports disaster took place under a full moon: 328 people died during a riot following a soccer game in Lima, Peru, on May 24, 1964.

□ Julius Caesar, Leon Trotsky, Alexander II (Russia), Francisco Madero (Mexican President), and Rafael Trujillo Molina (Dictator of Dominico) were all assassinated during full moon phases.

□ More people jump off the Golden Gate Bridge in San Francisco during full moons than at other times of the lunar month.

□ A study of suicides in France between 1842 and 1846 showed that most occurred during the full moon.

□ Several studies of suicides have shown significant increases when the moon is closest and farthest from the Earth (known as the perigee and apogee). These points in the moon's orbit do not always coincide with the times of full and new moons.

□ A study of tuberculosis deaths showed that the highest mortality rate occurred just after the full moon.

□ According to a 43-year study conducted at a lunatic asylum in England in the mid-1800s, most deaths at the asylum occurred during full moons.

A tornado which struck Venice, Italy, in 1970 killed thirty-five people.

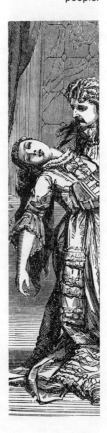

_____SPONTANEOUS COMBUSTION

"Death to intelligence, and long live death."
— General Millan-Astray

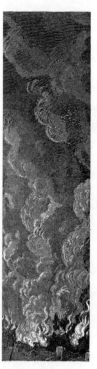

The most deadly earthquake in modern times was on July 28, 1976, in China; over 242,000 died.

There have been more than 200 recorded cases of people bursting into flame with no apparent cause, from the time of the first medical reporting in the 1600s. This phenomenon, known as spontaneous human combustion, has no acceptable scientific explanation, and is usually considered too far-fetched to be true by pragmatic investigators. Still, there are numerous witnessed accounts of people bursting into flame.

One of the most thorough investigations of human combustion involved the death of Mary Reeser, a 67-year-old widow in St. Petersburg, Florida. The remains of her body were discovered in her apartment on July 2, 1951. She had been almost obliterated by a fire that had burned the chair she was sitting in and a few square feet of the floor — but nothing else in the room. The body had been reduced from a weight of 175 pounds to less than 10 pounds of ash and other material. Arson investigators from the National Board of Underwriters, the FBI, and local experts were all mystified.

Tests conducted on animal tissue indicated that a source of heat in excess of 3000 degrees Fahrenheit would have been necessary to reduce a human body to such a state. But there was no possible explanation as to how such an enormous amount of heat could have been generated in an ordinary room without destroying everything in it.

The Reeser case is but one reported instance of spontaneous combustion. There are examples of combustion inside automobiles and within crowds of people. People have erupted into flames while walking and while sleeping. Combustion has occurred on isolated parts of the body, in all varieties of weather, and to people of all ages.

This strange condition has also been known to pop up in literature. In Herman Melville's *Redburn*, the crew of a ship find a sailor on fire: "Two threads of greenish fire, like a forked tongue, darted out between the lips and in a moment, the cadaverous face was covered by a swarm of wormlike flames . . . the uncovered body burned before us, precisely like a phosphorescent shark in a midnight sea."

Scraps of cloths and the tiny skeleton of a child missing since 1931 were discovered in an eagle's nest on a farm in eastern Finland in 1933. However, there has never been an authenticated report of an eagle actually attacking and carrying off a child.

————POISONOUS ANIMALS IN THE U.S.

"Wild animals never kill for sport. Man is the only one to whom the torture and death of his fellow creatures is amusing in itself."
— James A. Froude

Reports from Zambia recounted the deaths of nine people on the Namwala River in 1969 after their boats had been overturned by rampaging hippopotamuses.

☐ **Rattlesnake**: 6 deaths per year (The estimated mortality rate from all rattlesnake bites is about 2 percent.)
☐ **Insects** (unidentified): 6 per year
☐ **Wasps**: 5 per year
☐ **Bees**: 5 per year
☐ **Snakes** (unidentified): 4 per year
☐ **Yellowjackets**: 2 per year
☐ **Spiders** (unidentified): 2 per year
☐ **Scorpions**: 1 per year

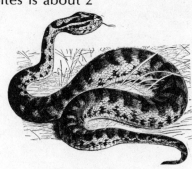

The only recorded fatality caused by a swan was from 1938, when a child was attacked by a swan and drowned in Methuen, Massachusetts.

☐ **Ticks**: 1 per year
☐ **Black widow spiders**: 1 every 2 years (There have been less than 75 recorded deaths since 1726.)
☐ **Brown spiders**: 1 every 2 years
☐ **Copperheads**: 1 every 3 years
☐ **Hornets**: 1 every 4 years
☐ **Water moccasins**: 1 every 8 years
☐ **Coral snakes**: 1 every 8 years
☐ **Ants**: 1 every 10 years
☐ **Snake serum**: 1 every 10 years
☐ **Portuguese Man-of-War**: 1 every 10 years
☐ **Gila monsters**: a total of eight deaths on record

(Most of the animals listed here cause deaths from anaphylactic shock. To those not susceptible, the bites or stings from these animals are usually not considered lethal or even dangerous.)

No verified reports exist of a human fatality from a giant clam, despite its image as perpetuated in the cinema.

The first known fatality from a captive tiger was Helen Bright, whose head was crushed by a tiger in England in 1850.

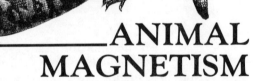

ANIMAL MAGNETISM

"Ideal mankind would abolish death, multiply itself million upon million, rear up city upon city, save every parasite alive, until the accumulation of mere existence is swollen to a horror."
— D. H. Lawrence

CATS

The domestic feline is of little danger to man, although persistent rumors claim that sleeping babies have been smothered by these popular pets.

Larger members of the cat family, however, do not pose such an imaginary danger. Hundreds of people have been devoured by leopards in Asia. Records show that in India alone, these large cats killed 125 people in the period from 1918-1926; an additional 350 victims were added to the list from 1959 to 1962.

Tigers are just as dangerous as leopards. When a tiger turns to humans for meat, it will often kill dozens of people before it is destroyed. Many tales of human-killing sprees by tigers have been recorded in Sumatra, India, and in other parts of southeast Asia.

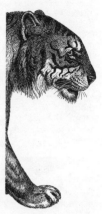

Lions in Africa, particularly young lions, have also been known to be man-eaters: there are recorded instances of dozens of victims being bagged by a single rogue cat. Though the incidents are less frequent on the American continent, jaguars and mountain lions have occasionally killed humans.

CANINES

Dogs may be man's best friend, but the same distinction does not apply to the dog's relative, the wolf. Wolves are not always vicious, but in recent history there have been a few validated reports of wolves attacking and killing men. In Europe and Asia, reports of attacks are more frequent and gruesome than elsewhere, suggesting that wolves on those continents are more aggressive and predatory toward humans. One Russian report of wolf attacks in 1875 totaled 161 victims for that year.

Other members of the canine family are rarely vicious towards humans. However, every year there are instances of domestic dogs killing people in the U.S. — mostly children.

Between 1959 and 1962, leopards killed at least 350 people in Asia.

Elephants on a rampage killed tweny-four people in India on July 10, 1972.

BEARS

Grizzly bears and polar bears are both extremely aggressive and ferocious as evidenced by the death tolls attributed to them. Hundreds of hunters, hikers, and campers have been killed by these fierce creatures since the North American continent was first explored. Along with the smaller American black bear, the grizzly and the polar bear add new victims to the list every year.

In recent years, in separate instances, a moose destroyed a boat carrying six men, killing two of them, and another moose attacked a car, killing the driver.

CROCODILES

These fearsome creatures account for an unverifiable number of deaths each year, but the total is probably about several hundred. A bizarre crocodile massacre took place in February, 1945, during World War II. In the Bay of Bengal, British troops forced Japanese troops to retreat into a swamp, and sealed off all the escape routes. Weapons fired from both sides apparently drove the resident crocodiles into the water, where they homed in on the blood of the wounded Japanese soldiers. After a night of being trapped with these creatures, only twenty of the 1,000 Japanese soldiers survived. Although British weapons and the environment of the swamp certainly added to the fatality rate, the crocodiles did more than their share to aid the war effort.

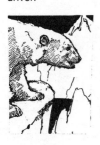

In February, 1982, a whale destroyed a small boat filled with people who were whale-watching in Baja California, Mexico. One of the passengers in the boat suffered a heart attack and died; several others were injured in the attack.

BARRACUDAS AND PIRANHAS

Few reports exist of fatalities from attacks by these fish. They are, nevertheless, definitely dangerous to humans.

STINGRAYS

Although many people are stung by these animals, only a few have ever been known to die as a result. Two of these fatalities were caused by the stingray spine being driven into the victims' hearts.

MOLLUSKS

This venomous cone shell, found in the Pacific Ocean, is known to have killed at least five divers, and perhaps as many as ten. Its venom is deadlier than that of either the rattlesnake or the common cobra.

ELECTRIC EELS

This bizarre denizen of South American rivers can generate and discharge more than 400 volts (at one ampere) — at a frequency of as much as 400 times per second. The charge can stun a large animal up to twenty feet away and contact with the fish is certain to be fatal. Although there are few recorded cases of fatalities, two workers were killed when they accidentally fell into a tank holding electric eels in Brazil in 1941.

Small parasitic catfish that are native to some parts of South America have a strong affinity for human urine — swimmers without the protection of clothing have had these fish swim up their urethas, with fatal results.

SNAKES

An estimated 30,000 to 40,000 people worldwide die each year from snake bites. The King Cobra is considered the most deadly of snakes, due to its size, the toxicity of its venom, and its general disposition toward humans. Be that as it may, the snake responsible for the most deaths is the

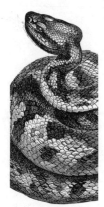

A murder case was solved in Australia in 1935 through the identification of an arm regurgitated from a captured shark. The arm had a recognizable tattoo, which led to the arrest of the murderer, who had apparently run out of room when packing his victim's body into a trunk. One arm was thrown into the sea and subsequently eaten by the shark. The case is known as the "Shark Arm Murder."

Common Cobra. An accounting of snake bite deaths:

☐ Japan: About 100 deaths a year from snake bite; most are caused by a snake similar to the Copperhead found in the U.S.

☐ Brazil: Anywhere from 2,000 to 4,000 deaths per year.

☐ Columbia: About 200 deaths per year.

☐ England: Fewer than ten deaths this century.

☐ Spain: About five deaths per year.

☐ Australia: About five deaths per year. (The Australian Death Adder is estimated to have a 50 percent fatality rate for its human victims; the American rattlesnake has about a 2 percent fatality rate.)

☐ Mexico: About 100-200 deaths per year. (Compare this to the more than 1,000 deaths attributed annually to scorpions.)

☐ Thailand: About 200 deaths per year.

☐ Burma: About 1,000 deaths per year (cobras).

☐ India: Anywhere from 10,000 to 20,000 deaths per year. (At least twelve varieties of snakes potentially lethal to man live in India.)

☐ Africa: Most parts of the continent experience fewer than thirty deaths per year.

SHARKS

Sharks are probably the most feared animal among humans. Sharks do kill people, but much of the fear is the product of sensational media reports. Until recently, no thorough statistical studies had been done to show exactly how dangerous these "monsters of the deep" really are. Recent analyses of shark attack information shows that on a world average, only 20 percent of the attack victims die. With an annual average of twenty attacks in the U.S., this produces an average of four deaths per year. The attacks peak in the morning hours, and are heaviest on weekends, when there is also the greatest number of people in the water.

Deaths from shark attacks are not always due to the severity of the wounds. In some cases they are the result of drowning, presumably because of panic or fainting. In fact, very few shark attacks produce wounds which are not treatable, and it is only the lack of proximity to emergency treatment which makes the attacks so lethal.

One of the significant results of shark attack studies points to the choice of victims — more than 90 percent have been male. Studies also show that the white shark and tiger shark are the two types most liable to attack, followed by the grey nurse shark and the nurse shark. Another recent study points to the probability that many, if not most, shark attacks on scuba divers and surfers occur because of the great visual similarity between them and the favorite natural food of sharks — sea lions.

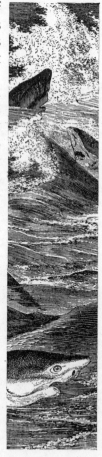

Few sharks are large enough to swallow a human body, but in one rare case, the body of a fully clothed teenage boy was found in the stomach of a captured shark in Japan in 1954.

Of the good samaritans who jumped to the rescue when others were attacked by sharks, there is only an estimated 1 percent fatality rate.

The most dangerous shark-infested area in the U.S. is the Atlantic coast of Florida, with the southern coast of California and the Gulf coast of Florida second deadliest. The safest place to swim is Connecticut.

*"Death is the only clear beautiful
conclusion of a great passion."*
— D. H. Lawrence

Chapter Nine

THE CALENDAR OF DEATH
A Daily Dose of Death

————————JANUARY

□ **JANUARY 1, 1953**: On his way to a concert date in Canton, Ohio, Hank Williams, twenty-nine-year-old singer and composer, dies of a heart attack in the back seat of a Cadillac. The driver discovers the death at a Puroil Gas Station in Oak Ridge, West Virginia. Earlier, near Rutledge, Tennessee, the driver had been stopped and ticketed for speeding by a policeman who commented that the person in the back seat looked dead.   □ **JANUARY 2, 1883**: Tom Thumb, dwarf General, dies.   □ **JANUARY 3, 1967**: Jack Ruby, convicted murderer of Lee Harvey Oswald, dies at the age of fifty-five in Parkland Memorial Hospital in Dallas. Cause of death: a blood clot in his lung.   □ **JANUARY 4, 1960**: Albert Camus, writer, dies when his Facel-Vega automobile runs off the road and strikes a tree. Camus was returning to Paris from the southern part of France. **1965**: T. S. Eliot, poet, dies in London, England.   □ **JANUARY 5, 1933**: Calvin Coolidge, twenty-ninth President of the U.S., dies of a heart attack on the floor of his bedroom in Northampton, Massachusetts. He is sixty years old at the time of his death. **1970**: Joseph Yablonski, of the United Mine Workers Union, and his wife and daughter are all shot to death at their home in Clarksville, Pennsylvania.   □ **JANUARY 6, 1919**: Theodore Roosevelt, twenty-sixth President of the U.S., dies from inflammatory rheumatism at Oyster Bay, New York, at the age of sixty. His last words: "Please put out the light." **1945**: Alexander Calder, sculptor, dies at age seventy-four in New York City.   □ **JANUARY 7, 1943**: Nicola Tesla, inventive genius, dies in New York City.   □ **JANUARY 8, 1642**: Galileo Galilei, astronomer, dies.   □ **JANUARY 9, 1923**: Katherine Mansfield, writer, dies in Fontainebleau, France. Her last words: "I believe I am going to die."   □ **JANUARY 10, 1645**: The Archbishop of Canterbury is beheaded at Tower Hill in London. **1951**: Sinclair Lewis, writer, dies surrounded by nuns in a sanitorium in Rome, Italy.   □ **JANUARY 11, 1928**: Thomas Hardy, writer, dies in Dorset, England.   □ **JANUARY 12, 1976**: Agatha Christie, mystery writer, dies.   □ **JANUARY 13, 1864**: Stephen Foster, composer, dies in a hospital in New York City, a few days after being found naked on the floor of his rented room in the Bowery. He left these words written on a scrap of paper: "Dear friends and gentle hearts." **1885**: Schuyler Colfax, seventeenth Vice President of the U.S., dies in Mankato, Minnesota, after walking between two railroad stations about a mile apart in thirty degree below zero weather. Local reports attribute his death to "fatal derangement of the heart's action." **1979**: Donny Hathaway, singer and arranger, commits suicide by jumping from the roof of the Essex House Hotel in New York City. □ **JANUARY 14, 1957**:   Humphrey Bogart, actor, dies. His last words, to Lauren Bacall: "Goodbye kid, hurry back." **1977**: Peter Finch, actor, dies. □ **JANUARY 15, 1867**:   In London, England, the ice on a Regent's Park lake gives way under a crowd of people; more than forty drown. **1919**: A huge holding tank containing more than two million gallons of molasses bursts open and sends a sea of the sticky substance through a large area of Boston, Massachusetts, hitting buildings and people with a wall of molasses twenty to thirty feet high. Twenty-one people die in the Great Boston Molasses Flood. □ **JANUARY 16, 1874**:   Chang and Eng, Siamese twins, die in Mount Airy, North Carolina. Chang dies first, followed about three hours later by Eng. **1935**: Ma Barker, outlaw gang leader, dies of a gunshot wound after a four-hour gun battle with police in Lake Welr, Florida. **1942**: Carole Lombard (born Jane Alice Peters), dies at the age of thirty-four in the crash of TWA flight #3, bound for Los Angeles from Indianapolis, Indiana. The plane crashes in the Table Rock Mountains, southeast of Las Vegas, Nevada, killing all twenty-two passengers, including Lombard's mother.   □ **JANUARY 17, 1893**: Rutherford B. Hayes, nineteenth President of the U.S., dies from heart disease at the age of seventy. **1977**: Gary Gilmore, convicted murderer, is executed by firing squad in Utah, marking an end of a ten-year ban on capital punishment in the U.S. □ **JANUARY 18, 1862**:   John Tyler, tenth President of the U.S., dies from "bilious fever" at the age of seventy-one .   His last words: "Doctor, I am going: perhaps it is best."   □ **JANUARY 19, 1907**: A railroad wreck in Fowler, Indiana, kills twenty-nine people.   □ **JANUARY 20, 1965**: Alan Freed, rock 'n roll disc jockey, dies in Palm Springs, Florida, of uremia. **1984**: Johnny Weissmuller, Olympic gold medal winner and screen star, dies from lung blockage at the age of seventy-nine.   □ **JANUARY 21, 1792**: Louis XVI is executed in Paris, France.   □ **JANUARY 22, 1879**: With only spears as weapons, Zulu warriors kill 1,745 British troops in the battle of Isandhlwana in southeast Africa. **1973**: Lyndon Johnson, thirty-sixth President of the U.S., dies at the San Antonio International Airport in Texas as he is being transported from his ranch to a hospital after suffering a heart attack.   □ **JANUARY 23, 1806**: William Pitt, Prime Minister of England, dies from typhoid. His last words: "Oh my country! How I love my country!" **1978**: Terry Kath, member of the rock group Chicago, dies while trying to prove a gun isn't loaded — by pointing it at his head and pulling the trigger.   ☐ **JANUARY 24, 1931**: Anna Pavlova, ballerina, dies of pleurisy of the lungs in The Hague, Holland. Her last words: "Get my swan costume ready." **1965**: Winston Churchill, British statesman, dies from cerebral thrombosis at the age of ninety in his home in London, England.   ☐ **JANUARY 25, 1881**: Fyodor Dostoyevsky, writer, dies a few days after suffering a hemorrhage that his doctor thought was not serious. His last words: "Hold me not back. My hour has come. I must die." **1947**: Alphonse "Scarface" Capone dies in Miami Beach, Florida. It is generally believed he died from an untreated, advanced case of syphilis.   ☐ **JANUARY 26, 1979**: Nelson Rockefeller, forty-first Vice-President of the U.S., dies of cardiac arrest at the age of seventy in New York City.   ☐ **JANUARY 27, 1851**: John James Audubon, wildlife artist, dies at the age of sixty-six, after living for several years in the shadow of senility. **1967**: While participating in a simulation of an upcoming launch, astronauts Virgil Grissom, Edward White, and Roger Chaffee die in a fire that sweeps through the capsule of the Apollo I spacecraft. ☐ **JANUARY 28, 1829**:   William Burke, body snatcher, is executed in Edinburgh, Scotland.   ☐ **JANUARY 29, 1933**: Scraps of cloth and the tiny skeleton of a child missing since 1931 are discovered in an eagle's nest on a farm in eastern Finland. **1977**: Freddie Prinze, comedian and actor, dies at the age of twenty-three in a Los Angeles hospital thirty-six hours after he had shot himself in the head with a revolver. A note found in his apartment said, "I cannot go on any longer."   ☐ **JANUARY 30, 1948**: Orville Wright, co-inventor of the airplane, dies of natural causes at the age of seventy-six in Dayton, Ohio. On the same day, three separate U.S. airplane crashes leave fifty people dead.   ☐ **JANUARY 31, 1956**: A. A. Milne, creator of *Winnie the Pooh*, dies in Hartfield, Sussex, England.

FEBRUARY

☐ **FEBRUARY 1, 1966**: Buster Keaton, film comedian, dies.   ☐ **FEBRUARY 2, 1895**: Frederick Douglass, social reformer, dies suddenly after dining with his wife. His last words: "Why, what does this mean?" **1970**: Bertrand Russell, philosopher, dies. **1979**: Sid Vicious, punk rocker, dies of a heroin overdose in New York City.   ☐ **FEBRUARY 3, 1889**: Belle Starr, outlaw, dies at the age of forty-one on a road near Eufaula, Oklahoma, the victim of an ambush. Inscribed on her tombstone: "Shed not for her the bitter tear/ Nor give the heart to vain regret/ 'Tis but the casket that lies here/ The gem that fills it sparkles yet." **1933**: Nine women, patients at a mental institution in Cleveland, Ohio, die in a fire that consumes the building where they are housed. Although the fire was discovered in time and the patients led to safety, they apparently found the night air too cold and their night clothes too thin — so they ran back inside to get warm by the fire. **1924**: Woodrow Wilson, twenty-seventh President of the U.S., dies of "apoplexy paralysis" in Washington, D.C., at the age of sixty-seven. **1959**: Ritchie Valens, "The Big Bopper", and Buddy Holly, die near Mason City, Iowa, in an airplane crash.   ☐ **FEBRUARY 4, 1976**:

Guatemala is hit by an earthquake that kills 22,836 people.   □ **FEBRUARY 5, 1889**: The ice on Pine Lake in Fulton County, New York, breaks; seven loggers drown.   □ **FEBRUARY 6, 1685**: Charles II of England dies the day after sixteen ounces of blood were bled from him. He had been suffering for several days from an unknown illness, which the royal physicians had been treating with most of the known "cures" of the time. **1951**: Eighty-four people die in a train wreck in Woodbridge, New Jersey.   □ **FEBRUARY 7, 1894**: Adolphe Sax, inventor of the saxophone, dies in Paris.   □ **FEBRUARY 8, 1933**: Mrs. Lucinda Mills, age sixty-seven, is strangled by her family during a religious ceremony inside her home near Tomahawk, Kentucky. **1936**: Charles Curtis, thirty-first Vice President of the U.S., dies in Washington, D.C.   □ **FEBRUARY 9, 1981**: Bill Haley, rock 'n roller, dies of a heart attack at age fifty-five in his home at Harlingen, Texas.   □ **FEBRUARY 10, 1912**: Joseph Lister, surgeon, dies at Walmer, Kent, England.   □ **FEBRUARY 11, 1933**: A little girl jumps more than 1,000 feet to her death into the crater of the Mihara Volcano on the island of Oshima in Japan. She is the first of fifty-six children to take the leap. The last jump is on May 9 — after which police guards are installed to prevent any more jumps.   □ **FEBRUARY 12, 1976**: Sal Mineo, actor, dies at the age of thirty-seven in Hollywood, California, after being stabbed by an unknown assailant.   □ **FEBRUARY 13, 1542**:   Catherine Howard, the fifth wife of Henry VIII of England, is beheaded. **1945**: American bombers saturate Dresden, Germany, with explosives on a series of raids that continue until February 15. The final death toll is more than 30,000.   □ **FEBRUARY 14, 1779**: Captain James Cook, explorer, dies at the hands of Hawaiian natives, with whom he had had a disagreement. He is stabbed and drowned, and his body rendered into pieces. Parts of Cook — his scalp, bare bones, and both hands preserved in salt — are returned to his crew. The remains are buried at sea. **1929**: Seven members of the North Side Gang in Chicago, Illinois, are murdered in a garage on North Clark Street in what comes to be called the St. Valentine's Day Massacre.   □ **FEBRUARY 15, 1856**:   Heinrich Heine, German poet, dies after suffering for years from an advanced case of syphilis. Days before he died, he told his wife, "God will forgive me — that's his job." **1981**: Michael Bloomfield, blues guitarist, dies of a suspected heroin overdose in his car in San Francisco, California. **1965**: Nat King Cole, singer, dies of lung cancer in Santa Monica, California.   □ **FEBRUARY 16, 1843**: A landslide in Troy, New York, kills eighteen people.   □ **FEBRUARY 17, 1934**: Albert I, King of Belgium, dies from a fall while mountain climbing. Shortly before, he had left this note for his climbing companions: "Follow the path for another fifty yards. I am going back to the foot of the rocks to make another climb. If I feel in good form, I shall take the difficult way up; if I do not, I shall take the easy one. I shall join you in an hour."   □ **FEBRUARY 18, 1933**: James "Gentleman Jim" Corbett, boxer, dies.   □ **FEBRUARY 19, 1942**:   Frank "The Dasher" Abbandando, dies in the electric chair. He received his nickname for allegedly dashing away from an intended victim so fast that he caught up to him from behind. Using his former pastime as a defense, his lawyer once defended him in court on a murder charge by claiming, "Ballplayers don't kill people."   □ FEBRUARY 20, 1725: First known scalping of Indians by white settlers takes place in New Hampshire. □ FEBRUARY 21, 1965:   Malcolm X, thirty-nine-year-old leader of the Black Nationalist movement, dies in an assassination attack in New York City. □ FEBRUARY 22, 1978:   Two railroad cars carrying liquid petroleum collide in Waverly, Tennessee. Fifteen people are killed when the leaking gas explodes two days later.   □ FEBRUARY 23, 1848: John Quincy Adams, sixth President of the U.S., dies in the Speaker's Room of the House of Representatives after suffering a heart attack. He is eighty years old. His last words: "This is the last of earth. I am content."   □ FEBRUARY 24, 1815: Robert Fulton, inventor of the steamboat, dies.   □ FEBRUARY 25, 1970: Mark Rothko, modernist painter, dies in New York City.   □ FEBRUARY 26, 1531: An earthquake in Lisbon, Spain, kills 20,000 people.   □ FEBRUARY 27, 1936: Ivan Pavlov, psychologist, dies in Leningrad, U.S.S.R.   □ FEBRUARY 28, 1966: Elliot See and Charles Bassett, astronauts, die in a plane crash on the roof of the Gemini Capsule building at the McDonnell Aircraft Company in St. Louis, Missouri. 1968: Frankie Lymon, lead singer with the Teenagers, dies from a heroin overdose in his grandmother's bathroom in New York City. □ FEBRUARY 29, 1960:   Melvin Purvis, FBI agent, commits suicide at the age of fifty-six at his home in Florence, South Carolina.

———————————MARCH

□ MARCH 1, 1910:   More than 100 people die in a landslide in Wellington, Washington.   □ MARCH 2, 1889: Several dogs, four calves, and a horse are electrocuted to demonstrate the effectiveness of electricity for executions. □ MARCH 3, 1960:   Leonard Warren, operatic baritone, dies during an ovation at the Metropolitan Opera in New York City. He had just finished an aria from Verdi's opera La Forza del Destino.   □ MARCH 4, 1963: William Carlos Williams, writer, dies in Rutherford, New Jersey.   □ MARCH 5, 1770: Seven residents of Boston, Massachusetts, are killed by British soldiers. The event has been commemorated as the Boston Massacre.   □ MARCH 6, 1836: The Alamo falls to Mexican army forces. The Texas side loses 187 men. 1932: John Philip Sousa, the March King, dies of a heart attack in a hotel room in Reading, Pennsylvania.   □ MARCH 7, 1913: Dynamite explodes in Baltimore, Maryland, killing fifty-five people.   □ MARCH 8, 1874: Millard Fillmore, thirteenth President of the U.S., dies in Buffalo, New York, at the age of seventy-four, suffering from paralysis and debility.   His last words: "The nourishment is palatable." 1930: William H. Taft, twenty-seventh President of the U.S., dies of debility at the age of seventy-two in Washington, D.C. □ MARCH 9, 1274:   After being struck on the head and knocked off his donkey by a low-hanging tree limb, saint Thomas Aquinas dies on the road to the Council of Lyons. According to legend, the donkey also died — from sorrow. 1916: Pancho Villa and 1,500 Mexican guerrillas attack Columbus, New Mexico, and kill seventeen American citizens. 1945: The most destructive air raid in history: the U.S. Army Air Corps destroys more than sixteen square miles of Tokyo in a nighttime incendiary bomb attack. The Corps use 334 B-29 bombers to drop 2,000 tons of bombs, which burn 250,000 buildings. The official death count on the ground is 83,793 fatalities, with an unofficial estimate of more than 100,000.   □ **MARCH 10, 1913**: Harriet Tubman, ex-slave and abolitionist, dies in Auburn, New York, at the Harriet Tubman Home for Aged Negroes, which she founded.   □ **MARCH 11, 1948**: Zelda Sayre Fitzgerald, the wife of F. Scott Fitzgerald, dies in a fire in an Asheville, North Carolina, mental hospital where she is a patient. Eight other women patients die in the same blaze. **1970**: Erle Stanley Gardner, age eighty, dies in Temecula, California.   □ **MARCH 12, 1926**: Edward Scripps, newspaperman, dies on board a ship off the coast of Liberia.   □ **MARCH 13, 1901**: Benjamin Harrison, twenty-third President of the U.S., dies of pneumonia at the age of sixty-seven in Indianapolis, Indiana. His last words: "Are the doctors here?" **1955**: Charlie Parker, jazz saxophonist, dies at age thirty-three in New York City. The coroner estimates the age of the body at fifty to sixty years old. Four possible causes of death — stomach ulcers, pneumonia, heart attack, and advanced cirrhosis — are suggested, but the death certificate lists lobar pneumonia. **1964**: Kitty Genovese, age twenty-eight, dies in the street in Queens, New York, after being stabbed repeatedly in front of thirty-seven witnesses, none of whom do anything to stop her attacker. **1968**: More than 6,400 sheep are reported to have been killed by nerve gas escaping from an Army test at Dugway Proving Grounds in Utah.   □ **MARCH 14, 1883**: Karl Marx dies. He once said, "Last words are for fools who haven't said enough." **1891**: Eleven Sicilian immigrants who had been indicted for the murder of the Chief of Police of New Orleans are lynched by a mob.   □ **MARCH 15, 44 B.C.**: Julius Caesar is assassinated. □ **MARCH 16, 1940**:   The Germans attack the Orkney Islands in Great Britain, killing one person. This is the first civilian death from an air raid in World War II. **1968**: My Lai Massacre: 109 Vietnamese men, women, and children are killed during a raid on their village by U.S. Army's Charlie Company, 1st Battalion, 20th Infantry, led by 1st Lieutenant William L. Calley.   □ **MARCH 17, 1886**: In Carrollton, Mississippi, a mob of white men shoot ten black men after removing them from a jail where they were awaiting trial for wounding a white man.   □ **MARCH 18, 1584**: Ivan the Terrible, Czar of Russia, dies while playing chess. The cause of death is said to be related to an unknown ailment that caused him "grievously to swell in the cods." **1965**: Farouk I, exiled King of Egypt, dies in Italy two hours after eating a dozen oysters, a leg of lamb, fried potatoes, beans, two oranges; drinking two bottles of Coca-Cola, a bottle of ginger soda, a glass of mineral water; and smoking a Havana cigar. □ **MARCH 19, 1950**:   Edgar Rice Burroughs, writer, dies.   □ **MARCH 20, 1933**: Guiseppe Zangara, age thirty-two, is electrocuted at the state prison in Florida for the shooting death of Mayor Anton Cermak of Chicago. Zangara shot Cermak and four others in a botched assassination attempt on the life of President-elect Franklin D. Roosevelt on February 15, 1933, in Miami, Florida. The assassin claimed to have had stomach pains for years which made him hate presidents and kings. At his trial, he was sentenced to eighty years hard labor for attempted murder (he told the judge, "Don't be stingy, give me 100 years."), and condemned to death for the murder of Chicago's mayor. □ **MARCH 21, 1617**:   Pocahontas, Powhatan Indian, dies in London, England, as she is preparing to return to America. She is buried at Gravesend, England. **1958**: Michael Todd, film producer, dies at the age of forty-nine in a plane crash about 35 miles southwest of Grants, New Mexico.   □ **MARCH 22, 1820**: Stephen Decatur, war hero, is shot and killed in a duel. **1978**: Karl Wallenda, aerialist, falls from a wire suspended 123 feet in the air between two hotels in San Juan, Puerto Rico, and dies instantly. He is seventy-three years old at the time of his death.   □ **MARCH 23, 1894**: A dynamite explosion at the Acme Powder Company in Black Run, Pennsylvania, kills five people.   □ **MARCH 24, 1882**: Henry Wadsworth Longfellow, poet, dies in Cambridge, Massachusetts. His last words, to his sister: "Now I know that I must be very ill, since you have been sent for." **1905**: Jules Verne, writer, dies in Amiens, France.   □ **MARCH 25, 1892**: Walt Whitman dies. Earlier, he had said, "Last words are not samples of the best which involve vitality at its full, and balance and perfect control scope. But they are valuable beyond measure to confirm and endorse the varied train, facts, theories and faith of the whole preceding life."   □ **MARCH 26, 1827**: Beethoven dies in Vienna as thunder and lightning strike the city. His last words: "Too bad! Too bad! It's too late!" **1945**: The fighting is finally over on Iwo Jima. The death toll stands at 6,821 Marines (including twelve Medal of Honor recipients).   □ **MARCH 27, 1945**: The last German V-2 rocket hits England, landing in Orpington, Kent, at 4:54 P.M. and killing one person. **1964**: A severe earthquake in Alaska kills 117 people. □ **MARCH 28, 1941**:   Virginia Woolf kills herself by placing a heavy rock in the pocket of her coat and walking into the River Ouse in England. **1968**: Yuri Gargarin, Soviet cosmonaut, dies in a plane crash. **1969**: Dwight D. Eisenhower, thirty-fourth President of the U.S., dies from heart disease at the age of seventy-eight. His last words: "I've always loved my wife. I've always loved my children. I've always loved my grandchildren. And I have always loved my country."   □ **MARCH 29, 1848**: John Jacob Astor, millionaire, dies. **1945**: The last German V-1 flying bomb is launched against England and destroyed in the air over Sittingbourne, Kent. A total of 9,200 V-1s were launched toward England, with more than half malfunctioning or being destroyed before hitting a target. The death toll from the bombs was 6,139, giving the bombs a final score of 1.5 deaths per unit.   □ **MARCH 30, 1967**: A Delta Airlines DC-8 crashes into a motel in New Orleans, Louisiana, killing eighteen people. □ **MARCH 31, 1850**:   John C. Calhoun, seventh Vice President of the U.S., dies in Washington, D.C. **1913**: John Pierpont Morgan, banker, dies in Rome, Italy.

APRIL

□ **APRIL 1, 1917**· Scott Joplin, composer, dies. **1950**: Dr. Charles Drew, the doctor responsible for developing plasma, dies after being in an automobile crash near Burlington, North Carolina. A still unsubstantiated story was circulated at the time claiming he was refused admission to a local hospital after the accident because he was black and subsequently, died from lack of blood.   □ **APRIL 2, 1893**: A tornado kills 100 people in Oklahoma.   □ **APRIL 3, 1882**: Jesse James, outlaw, age thirty-four, dies from a bullet to the back of his head. He is shot while standing on a chair to straighten a picture in his house in St. Joseph, Missouri.   □ **APRIL 4, 1841**: William Henry Harrison, ninth President of the U. S., dies at the age of sixty-eight. A month earlier, the President caught pneumonia at his inauguration where he delivered his speech in a cold drizzle — without a hat or overcoat. His last words: "Sir, I wish you to understand the true principles of government. I wish them carried out. I ask nothing more."   □ **APRIL 5, 1976**: Howard Hughes, billionaire, dies of kidney failure en route to a hospital in Houston, Texas. He is seventy years old at the time of his death.   □ **APRIL 6, 1971**: Igor Stravinsky, composer, dies in New York City.   □ **APRIL 7, 1739**: Richard Turpin, the "Highwayman," is executed.   □ **APRIL 8, 1887**: The Charity Hospital of Louisiana in New Orleans records the death of a forty-five-year-old patient, listing masturbation as the cause. **1973**: Pablo Picasso, artist, dies in France. Earlier, he had said, "Death holds no fear for me. It has a kind of beauty. What I am afraid of is falling ill and not being able to work. That's lost time."   □ **APRIL 9, 1976**: Phil Ochs, thirty-six-year-old folk singer, commits suicide by hanging himself in a closet at his sister's house.   □ **APRIL 10, 1963**: The U.S. nuclear-powered submarine _Thresher_ and all of its 129 crew members are lost during a practice dive about 200 miles east of Boston, Massachusetts.   □ **APRIL 11, 1926**: Luther Burbank, horticulturalist, dies in Santa Rosa, California, at the age of seventy-six.   □ **APRIL 12, 1945**: President Franklin Delano Roosevelt suffers a cerebral hemorrhage in Warm Springs, Georgia, and dies at the age of sixty-three. Earlier that day, he had torn up his draft card and remarked that he wouldn't be needing it any more. His last words: "I have a terrific headache."   □ **APRIL 13, 1917**: "Diamond Jim" Brady, financier, dies in Atlantic City, New Jersey, after several years of ill health that was linked to his tremendous appetite. □ **APRIL 14, 1912**: ·The _Titantic_ hits an iceberg in the Atlantic Ocean and sinks, causing the death of more than 1,500 people on board.   □ **APRIL 15, 1865**: Abraham Lincoln, sixteenth President of the U.S., dies after being shot by John Wilkes Booth at the Ford Theater. He is fifty-six years.   □ **APRIL 16, 69**: Marcus Salvius Otho, Emperor of Rome, commits suicide. **1879**: Saint Bernadette dies.   □ **APRIL 17, 1790**: Benjamin Franklin dies in Philadelphia, Pennsylvania. His last words: "A dying man can do nothing easy." **1945**: Ernie Pyle, American war correspondent, is killed by a Japanese sniper on Ie Island. Pyle is forty-four years old.   □ **APRIL 18, 1853**: William Rufus De Vane King, thirteenth Vice President of the U.S., dies in Cahaba, Alabama, of tuberculosis — although alcoholism probably was a contributing factor. In his last political campaign, he had been labelled "a hero of many a well-fought bottle." At the time of inauguration, he was in Havana, Cuba, too sick to return to

Washington. An Act of Congress allowed the oath of office to be administered there, making King the only executive officer of the U.S. to be sworn into office in a foreign country. **1955**: Albert Einstein, physicist, dies in Princeton, New Jersey, at the age of seventy-five.   ☐ **APRIL 19, 1882**: Charles Darwin dies from heart trouble. His last words: "I am not the least afraid to die." **1967**: Konrad Adenauer, ex-Chancellor of West Germany, dies from the effects of influenza in his home in West Germany, at the age of ninety-one.   ☐ **APRIL 20, 1812**: George Clinton, fourth Vice President of the U.S., dies in Washington, D.C., of pneumonia and "the general decay of Nature." **1875**: On board the American ship, *Jefferson Borden*, two mates are killed during a mutiny by the crew. The uprising is eventually suppressed.   ☐ **APRIL 21, 1910**: Mark Twain, writer, dies in Redding, Connecticut, at the age of seventy-five. Earlier, when a premature notice of his death had been published in a newspaper, he had said, "Rumors of my death are greatly exaggerated." ☐ **APRIL 22, 1915**:   The first deaths from gas warfare — used by the Germans on Europe's Western Front — are recorded.   ☐ **APRIL 23, 1616**: William Shakespeare, dramatist, dies in Stratford-upon-Avon, England. **1951**: Charles G. Dawes, the thirtieth Vice President of the U.S., dies in Evanston, Illinois. ☐ **APRIL 24, 1967**:   Vladimir Komarov, Soviet cosmonaut, dies during the re-entry of his space capsule. His parachute becomes tangled with the capsule and falls 4.3 miles to the surface of the earth. He becomes the first person to die during the execution of a space mission.   ☐ **APRIL 25, 1928**: Frank Lockhart, race car driver and winner of the Indianapolis 500, dies at the age of twenty-six at Daytona Beach, Florida, while trying to set a new world land speed record. He is driving at 225 miles per hour when a seashell causes a tire on his Stutz racer to blow, spinning the car end over end and ejecting the driver to his death.   ☐ **APRIL 26, 1901**: "Black Jack" Ketchum, train robber, dies on the gallows in Santa Fe, New Mexico. Due to the incorrect way the noose was placed around his neck and the weights tied to his body, he was decapitated when the hanging occurred. **1937**: At the invitation of Francisco Franco, the German Air Force experiments with aerial saturation bombing on the Spanish city of Guernica. The bombing takes place at noon on market day, killing 1,654 people (24 percent of the population). This was the first example of terror bombing in history. **1970**: Gypsy Rose Lee dies at the age of fifty-six in Los Angeles, California.   ☐ **APRIL 27, 1865**: The worst marine disaster in U.S. history: the steamer *Sultana* explodes on the Mississippi River, killing 1,700 passengers, mostly Union soldiers returning from Confederate prison camps. **1870**: The floor of the Supreme Court building in Richmond, Vermont, collapses and kills sixty-one people. **1932**: Hart Crane, writer, jumps over the side of a ship while traveling from Mexico to the U.S. He is wearing his pajamas. ☐ **APRIL 28, 1945**:   After a brief trial, Benito Mussolini, the dictator of Italy during most of World War II, is shot by anti-fascist partisans. He had been caught trying to escape to Switzerland on April 26.   ☐ **APRIL 29, 1887**: Twenty people die during a violent spring storm in Prescott County, Kansas. ☐ **APRIL 30, 1926**:   William Henry Jackson, the original "Zippy the Pinhead," dies in New York City after sixty-seven years in show business. **1945:** Adolf Hitler, German Reichsfuehrer, commits suicide in a bunker in Berlin. He is fifty-six at the time. **1956:** Alben W. Barkley, thirty-fifth Vice President of the U.S., dies in Lexington, Virginia, while giving a speech at Washington and Lee University. His last words were, "I would rather be a servant in the House of the Lord than to sit in the seats of the mighty."

MAY

□ **MAY 1, 1898:**   In the Spanish-American War battle of Manila Bay, American ships virtually destroy the Spanish fleet — killing 381 Spanish sailors without losing one American.   □ **MAY 2, 1960:** Caryl Chessman, the convicted "Redlight Bandit," dies in the gas chamber at San Quentin Prison in California. With appeals, he had been able to delay his execution for twelve years. **1972:** J.Edgar Hoover, director of the FBI, dies in his sleep at the age of seventy-seven in Washington, D.C.   □ **MAY 3, 1972:** Seven office workers die at their desks when a steam pipe explodes on the 36th floor of a skyscraper in New York City.   □ **MAY 4, 1970:** Four students die at Kent State University in Ohio during a confrontation with 100 National Guardsmen.   □ **MAY 5, 1821:** Napoleon Bonaparte dies. His last words: "France! Army! Head of the army! Josephine!"   □ **MAY 6, 1862:** Henry David Thoreau, dies in Concord, Massachusetts, after battling tuberculosis for several years. His last words: "Moose, Indian." **1937:** The German dirigible *Hindenberg* explodes while docking at Lakehurst, New Jersey; the thirty-six people on board are killed. □ **MAY 7, 1915:**   The *Lusitania* sinks off the coast of Ireland after being torpedoed by a German U-boat. About 2,000 people die.   □ **MAY 8, 1876:** Truganini, the last aborigine from Tasmania, dies.   □ **MAY 9 The** *John L. Avery*, a side-wheel river boat, sinks near Fort Adams, Mississippi, after hitting a snag on the Mississippi River. Seventy-five people drown.   □ **MAY 10, 1818:** Paul Revere, silversmith and patriot, dies in Boston, Massachusetts, at the age of eighty-two. **1863:** General Thomas "Stonewall" Jackson dies after contracting pneumonia while recovering from a wound received accidentally from his own army at the battle of Chancellorsville. **1977:** Joan Crawford dies in her apartment after several years of illness. She had refused diagnosis or treatment because of her faith in Christian Science. Her last words, upon hearing her housekeeper praying: "Damn it — don't you dare ask God to help me."   □ **MAY 11, 1981:** Bob Marley, reggae singer and composer, dies of cancer at age thirty-six in Cedars of Lebanon Hospital in Miami, Florida. □ **MAY 12, 1973:**   The last person executed with a guillotine in France goes under the blade.   □ **MAY 13, 1961:** Gary Cooper, actor, dies in Hollywood, California, at the age of sixty.   □ **MAY 14, 1970:** Two students die during a confrontation with police at Jackson State College in Mississippi.   □ **MAY 15, 1886:** Emily Dickinson, poet, dies at the age of fifty-six in Amherst, Massachusetts.   □ **MAY 16, 1873:** A dam break on the Mills River in Massachusetts causes 144 deaths downstream in Williamsburg, Leeds, and

Haydensville. **1920**: Levi Parsons Morton, twenty-second Vice President of the U.S., dies on his birthday in Rhinebeck, New York. ☐ **MAY 17, 1875**: John Cabell Breckenridge, fourteenth Vice President of the U.S., dies in Lexington, Kentucky, from liver problems. **1974**: Six members of the Symbionese Liberation Army die in a gun battle with police in Los Angeles, California. ☐ **MAY 18, 1980**:   Mt. St. Helens erupts in Washington State, killing fourteen people.   ☐ **MAY 19, 1935**: Thomas Edward Lawrence (of Arabia) dies in a motorcycle accident in England.   ☐ **MAY 20, 1946**: An Army C-45 airplane crashes into the 58th floor of the Manhattan Building in New York City; five people are killed.   ☐ **MAY 21, 1952**: John Garfield, actor, dies of a heart attack at age thirty-nine in a New York City apartment.   ☐ **MAY 22, 1949**: James Forrestal, who had resigned as the Secretary of Defense of the U.S. only a few days previously, dies as the result of a leap from the 16th floor window of the National Naval Medical Center in Bethesda, Maryland. He is fifty-seven years old at the time, and a victim of a sudden mental and physical collapse. A note quoting Sophocles on the subject of death is found in his hospital room. ☐ **MAY 23, 1934**:   Bonnie and Clyde die in a police ambush in which they receive twenty-three and twenty-five bullet wounds, respectively. Bonnie is twenty-three years old at the time, and Clyde is twenty-five. **1701**: Captain William Kidd, pirate, dies on the gallows in London, England.   ☐ **MAY 24, 1913**: A pier in Long Beach, California, collapses, killing thirty-five people. ☐ **MAY 25, 1979**:   An American Airlines DC-10 crashes near O'Hare Airport in Chicago, Illinois, killing 272 people on the plane and three on the ground. ☐ **MAY 26, 1868**:   The last public execution takes place in England with the hanging of Michael Barrett, convicted of complicity in the deaths of thirteen people.   ☐ **MAY 27, 1964**: Jawaharlal Nehru, the Prime Minister of India, dies at the age of seventy-four. The cause of death is listed as a heart attack. ☐ **MAY 28, 1972**:   The Duke of Windsor, ex-King of England, dies of cancer at the age of seventy-seven at his home in Paris, France.   ☐ **MAY 29, 1911**: W. S. Gilbert, playwright, dies of a heart attack while trying to rescue a young female guest who is swimming with him in his private lake. He is seventy-four. **1942**: John Barrymore, actor, dies at the Presbyterian Hospital in Hollywood, California, at the age of fifty-nine. Causes of death are listed as myocarditis, chronic nephritis, cirrhosis of the liver, and gastric ulcers.   ☐ **MAY 30, 1972**: The Lod Airport Massacre: after getting off a plane from Paris, France, three terrorists from Japan, using machine guns and hand grenades, kill twenty-eight people at the Tel Aviv airport.   ☐ **MAY 31, 1889**: Rushing waters of the Conemaugh River in Pennsylvania take the lives of 2,295 people. The disaster becomes known as the Johnston Flood. **1962**: Adolf Eichmann, convicted Nazi war criminal, is hanged in Ramale, Israel. He is fifty-six years old at the time of his execution.

JUNE

☐ **JUNE 1, 1868**:   James Buchanan, fifteenth President of the U.S., dies of rheumatic gout in Lancaster, Pennsylvania, at the age of seventy-seven. His last words: "O Lord, God Almighty, as Thou wilt." **1925**: Thomas Riley Marshall, twenty-eighth Vice President of the U.S., dies in Washington, D.C. **1968**: Helen Keller, age eighty-seven, dies from a stroke in Westport, Connecticut. □ **JUNE 2, 1941**:   Lou Gehrig, baseball player, dies of amyotrophic lateral sclerosis in New York City. This rare disease subsequently comes to be known as "Lou Gehrig's Disease."   □ **JUNE 3, 1953**: Billy Joe McAllister jumps off the Tallahatchee Bridge.   □ **JUNE 4, 1798**: Casanova, the legendary lover, dies in Bohemia· at the age of seventy-three. His last words: "I have lived as a philosopher and am dying a Christian." **1887**: William Almon Wheeler, nineteenth Vice President of the U.S., dies in Malone, New York. According to a report in a newspaper at the time, his life "went out so gradually and quietly that it was hard to mark the exact moment of its flight." **1918**: Charles W. Fairbanks, twenty-sixth Vice President of the U.S., dies in Indianapolis, Indiana, of intestinal nephritis. **1976**: The Teton Dam bursts in Idaho, killing eleven people.   □ **JUNE 5, 1900**: Stephen Crane, writer, dies of tuberculosis at the age of twenty-eight in Badenweiler, Germany.   □ **JUNE 6, 1968**: Robert Kennedy, U.S. Senator from New York, dies after hours of surgery at Good Samaritan Hospital. He had been shot by an assassin the day before in the Hotel Ambassador in Los Angeles, California.   □ **JUNE 7, 1937**: Jean Harlow (born Harlean Carpentier) dies from cholecystitis, an inflammation of the gall bladder, at age twenty-six in Los Angeles, California. Her mother, a Christian Scientist, would not allow medical treatment, so by the time that Harlow was brought to the hospital, the infection was out of control.   □ **JUNE 8, 1809**: Thomas Paine, author, dies in New York City. A few days before his death a visitor challenged his outspoken stance for atheism, to which he replied, "I have no wish to believe on that subject." **1845**: Andrew Jackson, seventh President of the U.S., dies at the Hermitage, in Nashville, Tennessee, at the age of seventy-eight, the victim of dropsy and consumption. His last words: "I hope to meet each of you in heaven. Be good children, all of you, and strive to be ready when the change comes." **1967**: The USS *Liberty*, a U.S. Navy ship, is attacked by Israeli torpedo boats and fighter planes in international waters north of the Sinai Peninsula. Thirty-four U.S. sailors die. Israel later apologizes for the attack, claiming it was accidental.   □ **JUNE 9, 1870**: Charles Dickens, author, dies at his country home in England at the age of fifty-eight. He had been in a coma since the day before, and had been suffering from partial paralysis for some time. **1893**: The Ford Theater collapses in Washington, D.C., killing twenty-two people. **1911**: Carry Nation, temperance leader, dies at the age of sixty-four in a hospital in Leavenworth, Kansas.   □ **JUNE 10, 1893**: Miss Fitzsimmons, kangaroo boxer, dies in Australia.   □ **JUNE 11, 1825**: Daniel D. Tompkins, sixth Vice President of the U.S., dies in Tompkinsville, New York, probably from the effects of excessive drinking. He had written that he suffered from, "toilsome days, sleepless nights, anxious cares, domestic bereavements, impaired constitution, debilitated body, unjust abuse and censure, and accumulated pecuniary embarrassments." **1937**: George

Gershwin dies of a brain tumor in Los Angeles, California. He is thirty-eight years old at the time of his death.   □ **JUNE 12, 1844**: Spanish soldiers execute Placido, a Cuban poet, for his involvement in the uprising of slaves. Ten other conspirators die with the first volley of shots, but Placido is only wounded, and calls for the soldiers to end his misery with a second volley — a request quickly granted. **1950**: Two Air France planes — on separate flights from Saigon to Paris — crash in the same area near Bahrein in the Persian Gulf. Forty-seven people die in one crash; forty in the other.   □ **JUNE 13, 323 B.C.**: Alexander the Great dies from a fever at the age of thirty-three.   □ **JUNE 14, 1801**: Benedict Arnold, traitor, dies in London, England. **1914**: Adlai Ewing Stevenson, twenty-third Vice President of the U.S., dies in Bloomington, Illinois.   □ **JUNE 15, 1849**: James Knox Polk, eleventh President of the U.S., dies at the age of fifty-three in Nashville, Tennessee. Diarrhea is listed as the cause of death. □ **JUNE 16, 1925**:   Fifty people die in a train wreck in Hackettstown, New Jersey.   □ **JUNE 17, 1850**: The steamer *Griffith* burns on Lake Erie, killing 300 people.   □ **JUNE 18, 1975**: Prince Museid is beheaded in Saudi Arabia for his part in the assassination of King Faisal.   □ **JUNE 19, 1972**: Hurricane Agnes comes ashore in Florida, beginning a ten-day excursion along the Atlantic coast. The final death toll is 118 people.   □ **JUNE 20, 1947**: "Bugsy" Siegel, gangster, dies from three rifle shots to the head in a mansion in Beverly Hills, California.   □ **JUNE 21, 1877**: Eight members of the Molly McGuires, an underground Irish protest group, are hanged in two Pennsylvania towns, Pottsville and Mauch Chunk. They had been found guilty of violent acts against the personnel and property of local coal mines.   □ **JUNE 22, 1969**: Judy Garland, actress, dies at the age of forty-seven in London, England, of a drug overdose.   □ **JUNE 23, 1922**: A labor riot in Herrin, Illinois, ends after several days, leaving thirty-six dead.   □ **JUNE 24, 1908**: Grover Cleveland, twenty-second President of the U.S., dies at the age of seventy-one in Princeton, New Jersey. The cause of death: debility and coronary sclerosis. His last words: "I have tried so hard to do right."   □ **JUNE 25, 1876**: At the Battle of the Little Bighorn, General George Armstrong Custer and 211 U.S. soldiers are killed by attacking Indians from various tribes, led by Sitting Bull.   □ **JUNE 26, 1976**: An earthquake in Indonesia kills more than 3,000 people.   □ **JUNE 27, 1844**: A mob breaks into the jail in Carthage, Illinois, and shoots Joseph Smith, Mormon leader. At the time of his death, he is being held on charges of arson, treason, and polygamy.   □ **JUNE 28, 1836**: James Madison, fourth President of the U.S., dies from debility at the age of eighty-five. His last words: "I always talk better lying down." **1968**: A man is killed after falling out of the door of a DC-3 airplane as it is flying 8,000 feet over southwest Missouri. He did not have a parachute.   □ **JUNE 29, 1967**: On her way to a television station, Jayne Mansfield, actress, dies in a automobile accident in New Orleans, Louisiana. Her car, traveling at high speeds, runs into the back of a truck and Mansfield is decapitated.   □ **JUNE 30, 1933**: Fatty Arbuckle, actor and director, dies of a heart attack in a hotel bed in New York City. **1974**: Alberta King, the mother of Dr. Martin Luther King, Jr., is shot and killed while playing the organ at the

Ebenezer Baptist Church in Atlanta, Georgia. She is sixty-nine years old at the time of her death.

JULY

□ **JULY 1, 1546:**   Martin Luther, religious reformer, dies in Germany. **1860:** Charles Goodyear, inventor, dies, $200,000 in debt, in New York City. **1884:** Allan Pinkerton, detective, dies in Chicago at the age of sixty-five. **1896:** Harriet Beecher Stowe, writer, dies in Hartford, Connecticut. **1904:** Anton Chekhov, author, dies in Germany, at the resort of Badenweiler at the age of forty-four. He had been suffering from tuberculosis for many years. **1976:** After undergoing several months of continuing exorcism by a Roman Catholic priest, Anneliese Michel, West German college student, dies at the age of twenty-three from malnutrition and dehydration. As a result of her death, the Church adds a requirement that a doctor always be present during exorcisms.
□ **JULY 2, 1961:**   Ernest Hemingway, writer, dies at his home in Ketchum, Idaho, of a self-inflicted shotgun wound.   □ **JULY 3, 1969:** While swimming alone and under the influence of drugs and alcohol, Brian Jones, one of the original members of the Rolling Stones, drowns in the pool at his home in England. He is twenty-five years old at the time. **1971:** Jim Morrison, singer and composer with The Doors, dies at the age of twenty-eight, in the bathtub of a hotel room in Paris, France. His death is attributed to heart failure; popular speculation blames an overdose of heroin.   □ **JULY 4, 1949:** A freak windstorm hits the eastern coast of the U.S. between New Jersey and southern New England, with gusts more than sixty miles per hour. Hundreds of small boats are capsized and nine people drown. **1826:** John Adams, second President of the U.S., dies of debility at the age of ninety. His last words: "Independence forever." He is buried in Quincy, Massachusetts. **1826:** Thomas Jefferson, third President of the U.S., dies of diarrhea at the age of eighty-three. His final words: "I resign my spirit to God, my daughter to my country." He is buried in Charlottesville, Virginia. **1831:** James Monroe, fifth President of the U.S., dies of debility at the age of seventy-three in New York City. He is buried in Richmond, Virginia. **1891:** Hannibal Hamlin, fifteenth Vice President of the U.S., dies in Bangor, Maine, from dyspepsia and heart problems.   □ **JULY 5, 1950:** The first U.S. soldier dies in the Korean War.
□ **JULY 6, 1893:**   Guy de Maupassant, writer, dies from an advanced case of syphilis at the age of forty-two. He had searched for years unsuccessfully for relief from pain; a year before his death, he wrote, "I am in my death agony. I have a softening of the brain brought on by bathing my nostrils with salt water. The salt has fermented in my brain, and every night my brains are dripping away through my nose and mouth in a sticky paste." **1944:** A fire during a performance at a Ringling Brothers and Barnum and Bailey Circus in Hartford, Connecticut, causes a panic inside the main tent. The stampede results in the deaths of 168 people.   □ **JULY 7, 1959:** While under arrest for narcotic addiction, "Lady Day" Billie Holliday, singer, dies at age forty-four in

Metropolitan Hospital in New York City.   □ **JULY 8, 1844**: An anti-Irish riot in Philadelphia, Pennsylvania, ends after several days of violence. The death toll reaches fifty.   □ **JULY 9, 1850**: Zachary Taylor, twelfth President of the U.S., dies in office, at the age of sixty-five. His death is caused by bilious fever, typhoid fever, and cholera. His last words: "I regret nothing, but am sorry that I am about to leave my friends." He is buried in Louisville, Kentucky.   □ **JULY 10, 1972**: In India, it is reported that elephants on a rampage attacked five villages and killed at least twenty-four people.   □ **JULY 11, 1804**: Alexander Hamilton is killed in a duel with Aaron Burr.   □ **JULY 12, 1942**: Max Geller, the owner of the Green Parrot Bar in New York City, is shot and killed during a robbery. None of the twenty customers in the bar at the time admit seeing the shooting. A police detective studies the case for several years and finally identifies the culprit with the help of the bar's resident parrot. The bird kept repeating the name of the murderer.   □ **JULY 13, 1863**: During a three-day riot in New York City, an estimated 2,000 people die. The riot begins in response to President Lincoln's plan to draft citizens into the army. The dead include at least 350 police and militiamen, as well as eighty-eight blacks, who were the object of racial hatred. Many of the victims — including at least one child — are axed to death, hanged from trees and lampposts, stoned, or burned alive in buildings.   □ **JULY 14, 1881**: Billy the Kid, outlaw, dies at the age of twenty-one from a shot fired by Pat Garrett, who was waiting in ambush in a dark room in Fort Sumner, New Mexico. **1966**: Eight student nurses die in their apartment in Chicago, Illinois, the victims of an attack by Richard Speck. Five are strangled and three are stabbed to death.   □ **JULY 15, 1793**: Jean Paul Marat, writer and revolutionary, dies in his bathtub from multiple knife wounds inflicted by a non-admirer. **1940**: Robert Wadlow, the tallest man in the world, dies at the age of twenty-two from a severe infection caused by the braces he wore to help him stand up. He is eight-feet, eleven-inches tall and weighs 491 pounds at the time of his death.   □ **JULY 16, 1965**: While walking near the U.S. Embassy in London, Adlai Stevenson, U.S. statesman, dies at the age of sixty-five from a heart attack.   □ **JULY 17, 1974**: A circus elephant chained to a tree in Oquawka, Illinois, is killed by lightning.   □ **JULY 18, 1817**: Jane Austin, novelist, dies in England from an ailment that was diagnosed by a medical historian in 1964 as Addison's disease. **1981**: At the Hyatt Regency Hotel in Kansas City, a walkway collapses, killing 110 people.   □ **JULY 19, 1969**: Mary Jo Kopechne dies of undetermined causes after the car in which she is riding with Senator Edward Kennedy plunges off a bridge on Chappaquiddick Island in Massachusetts.   □ **JULY 20, 1973**: Bruce Lee, actor, dies at the age of thirty-three in Hong Kong.   □ **JULY 21, 1880**: A flooding accident in a tunnel construction site underneath the Hudson River in New York kills twenty workers.   □ **JULY 22, 1869**: John Roebling, chief engineer for the construction of the Brooklyn Bridge, dies from a tetanus infection that set in after the toes on one of his feet were amputated in an accident on the bridge site. **1934**: John Dillinger, age thirty-one, receives multiple gunshot wounds in an FBI ambush. He dies outside the Biograph Theater in Chicago,

Illinois.   □ **JULY 23, 1885**: Ulysses S. Grant, eighteenth President of the U.S., dies at the age of sixty-three from carcinoma of the tongue and tonsils in Mt. McGregor, New York. His last word is, "Water."   □ **JULY 24, 1862**: Martin Van Buren, eighth President of the U.S., dies from asthma in Kinderhook, New York, at the age of seventy-nine. His last words: "There is but one reliance." **1974**: Cass Elliot, singer, dies at the age of thirty-three in London, England. Although popular reports had her choking to death on a ham sandwich, the official autopsy states that death was due to a heart attack brought on by an overweight condition.   □ **JULY 25, 1933**: In New York City, a distraught machinist dies in a closet after eating half of a roll he had poisoned while having dinner in a restaurant. The other half of the roll was snatched and eaten by a woman, who also died.   □ **JULY 26, 1863**: Sam Houston, Texas hero, dies in Huntsville, Texas, at the age of sixty-nine. His last words: "Texas, Texas." □ **JULY 27, 1852**:   During a race on the Hudson River near Yonkers, New York, the steamboat *Henry Clay* burns, killing seventy people. **1889**: A windstorm in Chicago, Illinois, causes the deaths of twenty people.   □ **JULY 28, 1540**: Thomas Cromwell is beheaded in London. **1945**: An Army B-25 bomber crashes into the side of the Empire State Building in New York City, 915 feet above the ground. Three people in the plane and ten people in the building are killed.   □ **JULY 29, 1967**: A fire breaks out on the U.S. aircraft carrier *Forrestal* in the Gulf of Tonkin off the coast of North Vietnam. The worst catastrophe in the Navy since World War II, the fire leaves 134 sailors dead. □ **JULY 30, 1784**:   Diderot, writer, dies after eating an apricot his wife had warned him not to eat. His final words: "How in the devil can it hurt me?" □ **JULY 31, 1875**:   Andrew Johnson, seventeenth President of the U.S., dies of paralysis at the age of sixty-six in Carter's Station, Tennessee. His last words: "Oh, do not cry. Be good children and we shall all meet in Heaven." He is buried in Greeneville, Tennessee.

AUGUST

□ **AUGUST 1, 1966**:   Charles Whitman, ex-Marine, dies at the age of twenty-four atop the Tower on the University of Texas Campus. Shot by an Austin, Texas policeman, Whitman had killed twenty people — including his wife and his mother — in a shooting spree.   □ **AUGUST 2, 1923**: Warren G. Harding, twenty-eighth President of the U.S., dies in a hotel in San Francisco after becoming ill, possibly from ptomaine poisoning in Grant's Pass, Oregon. He is fifty-seven years old at the time of his death. The final causes of death are determined to be a ruptured artery in the brain, pneumonia, enlargement of the heart, and high blood pressure. His last words: "Go on, read some more." **1876**: "Wild Bill" Hickok, age thirty-nine, dies of a gunshot in the back of his head while playing poker at Mann's Saloon Number 10 in Deadwood, Dakota Territory. Hickok was holding two pairs, aces and eights; thereafter this combination would be known as the "dead man's hand." **1979**: Thurman Munson, captain of the New York Yankees, dies when his private plane crashes after takeoff in Canton, Ohio. ☐ **AUGUST 3, 1903**: Martha "Calamity Jane" Cannary, age fifty, dies in a hotel bed in Terry, South Dakota. Her last words are, "Bury me next to Bill" (apparently referring to Wild Bill Hickok). **1966**: Lenny Bruce, comedian, dies at age forty-one of "acute morphine poisoning" in Hollywood, California. ☐ **AUGUST 4, 1892**: Lizzie Borden, of Fall River, Massachusetts, "gave her mother forty whacks, and when she was done, she gave her father forty-one." (The actual number of blows: nineteen for Mrs. Borden, and ten for Mr. Borden.) The accused is found innocent in court. ☐ **AUGUST 5, 1962**: Marilyn Monroe, thirty-six-year-old actress, dies of an apparent accidental overdose of barbiturates in her home in Hollywood, California. ☐ **AUGUST 6, 1890**: William Kemmler, ax murderer, becomes the first person to be executed in an electric chair. The execution takes place at Auburn Prison in New York. **1945**: Hiroshima, Japan is hit by an atomic bomb which kills about 78,000 people. ☐ **AUGUST 7, 1963**: Patrick Bouvier Kennedy, premature son born to President and Mrs. Kennedy, dies at the age of two days. ☐ **AUGUST 8, 1945**: Nagasaki, Japan is hit with an atomic bomb. More than 30,000 people are killed by the blast. ☐ **AUGUST 9, 1969**: Sharon Tate, actress, is murdered along with four friends at her home in Beverly Hills, California. Charles Manson and members of his "family" are later convicted of the crime. ☐ **AUGUST 10, 1932**: Rin Tin Tin dies. ☐ **AUGUST 11, 1956**: Jackson Pollock, artist, dies after losing control of the convertible he was driving near his home on Long Island, New York. When the car overturned, he was thrown out and struck a tree, causing a skull fracture and brain laceration. **1965**: The Watts riots begin in Los Angeles, California. The riots last for six days, during which time thirty-five people are killed. ☐ **AUGUST 12, 1827**: William Blake, artist and writer, dies after singing a song about heaven. A witness to the death said, "I have been at the death, not of a man, but of a blessed angel." ☐ **AUGUST 13, 1966**: Twenty-nine people die in a fire at a Salvation Army home in Melborne, Australia. This represents the worst body count from a fire in Australian history. ☐ **AUGUST 14, 1893**: Seven die in the Senate Hotel Fire in Chicago, Illinois. ☐ **AUGUST 15, 1935**: Will Rogers, humorist and actor, and Wiley Post, aviator, die in a plane crash near Point Barrow, Alaska. Rogers is fifty-six and Post thirty-six at the time of their deaths. ☐ **AUGUST 16, 1948**: George Herman "Babe" Ruth dies from cancer at the age of fifty-three in New York City. 1949: Margaret Mitchell, forty-nine-year-old author of *Gone With The Wind*, dies in a hospital in Atlanta, Georgia, where she was taken after being struck by a taxi. She was on her way to see a movie at the time. The cab driver is later convicted of involuntary manslaughter. **1977**: Elvis Presley, singer and actor, dies on the bathroom floor of his mansion, Graceland, in Tennessee. The forty-two-year-old entertainer was apparently the victim of misuse of drugs, although the autopsy report indicated death from natural causes. ☐ **AUGUST 17, 1915**: Leo Frank, factory manager, is lynched in Marietta, Georgia, after his death sentence is commuted to life imprisonment. Many believe that the lynching is related to his being Jewish. ☐ **AUGUST 18, 1227**: Genghis Khan, leader of the Mongol hordes, dies. **1976**: While pruning a tree

in the demilitarized zone, two U.S. soldiers are killed by North Korean soldiers.
□ **AUGUST 19, 1895**:   John Wesley Hardin, gunfighter and lawyer, dies at age forty-two from a gunshot in the back of the head while standing at a bar in El Paso, Texas. His nemesis, the local constable, claims that he shot in self-defense — as Hardin was able to see him in the mirror.   □ **AUGUST 20, 1940**: Leon Trotsky, exiled Russian leader, is murdered in Mexico.   □ **AUGUST 21, 1971**: George Jackson, a Black Panther and one of the Soledad Brothers, is shot and killed while attempting to escape from San Quentin Prison in California.
□ **AUGUST 22, 1922**:   Michael Collins, one of the founders of the I. R. A., is assassinated in Ireland.   □ **AUGUST 23, 1926**: Rudolph Valentino (born Rodolfo Alfonzo Rafaelo Pierre Filibert Guglielmi di Valentine d'Antonguolla), silent screen actor, dies at age thirty in New York City. The cause: blood poisoning from a perforated ulcer. **1927**: Nicola Sacco and Bartolomeo Vanzetti are executed in Massachusetts. Charged with armed robbery and murder, the pair are later cleared by proclamation. **1947**: Roy Chadwick, airplane designer, and three other passengers die in England immediately following the takeoff of a new plane Chadwick had designed. An investigation reveals that the aileron controls had been installed in reverse.   □ **AUGUST 24, 79**:   Pliny the Elder, Roman writer, dies after he approached Mount Vesuvius during its eruption in order to study the event. The apparent cause of death: inhalation of poisonous fumes.   □ **AUGUST 25, 1967**: Paul Muni, actor, dies at the age of seventy-two, from heart failure. His last words: "Papa, I'm hungry." **1967**. George Lincoln Rockwell, leader of the American Nazi Party, dies in his parked car outside a laundromat in Arlington, Virginia. He had been shot by another member of his Nazi organization.   □ **AUGUST 26, 1874**: Vigilantes forcibly remove sixteen blacks from a jail in Trenton, Tennessee, and shoot them.   □ **AUGUST 27, 1967**: Brian Epstein, record producer, dies at age thirty-three in London, England, of "accidental death through sleeping tablets."   □ **AUGUST 28, 1968**: John Gordon Mein, U.S. Ambassador to Guatemala, dies at the age of fifty-four in a rebel ambush, the first Ambassador killed while on duty.   □ **AUGUST 29, 1935**: Queen Astrid of Belgium dies in an automobile accident in Switzerland.   □ **AUGUST 30, 55 B.C.**: Cleopatra is bitten by an asp and dies.   □ **AUGUST 31, 1969**: Rocky Marciano, former heavyweight boxing champ, dies in a plane crash in Newton, Iowa.

SEPTEMBER

□ **SEPTEMBER 1, 1914**:   Martha, the last passenger pigeon in the world, dies in her cage at the Cincinnati Zoo.   □ **SEPTEMBER 2, 1894**: Twelve towns are destroyed and hundreds of people killed by forest fires in northwest Wisconsin.   □ **SEPTEMBER 3, 1875**: In Fort Smith, Arkansas, six convicted criminals are executed before a crowd of 5,000. The event becomes known as "The Dance of Death," and the judge responsible for the sentences earns the nickname, "Hanging" Parker.   □ **SEPTEMBER 4, 1965**: Albert Schweitzer, physician and musician, dies at the age of ninety in his hospital in Gabon.

Death is attributed to circulatory problems related to his age.   □ **SEPTEMBER 5, 1972**: Two members of the Israeli Olympic team die in their dormitory in Munich, West Germany, the victims of an attack by members of the "Black September" terrorist group. The next day, five terrorists and nine of their Israeli hostages die during a shootout with authorities.   □ **SEPTEMBER 6, 1971**: Separate lightning bolts in Macon County, Tennessee, and in Monroe County, Kentucky, each kill four workers inside tobacco sheds.   □ **SEPTEMBER 7, 1944**: A Japanese ship carrying American POWs is torpedoed by the submarine, USS *Barb*, killing 668.   □ **SEPTEMBER 8, 1900**: Galveston, Texas is hit by a hurricane. Between 6,000 and 7,000 people lose their lives. **1944**: The first German V-2 rocket hits England, near London, at 6:40 p.m. It kills two people.   □ **SEPTEMBER 9, 1976**: Mao Tse-tung, chairman of the Chinese Communist Party, dies of an undisclosed illness at the age of eighty-two in Peking.   □ **SEPTEMBER 10, 1962**: A U.S. Strategic Air Command plane crashes near Mount Kit Carson in Washington state, killing forty-four.   □ **SEPTEMBER 11, 1970**: A tornado hits Venice, Italy, killing thirty-five people. □ **SEPTEMBER 12, 1972**:   William Boyd, portrayer of "Hopalong Cassidy," dies.   □ **SEPTEMBER 13, 1899**: Henry Bliss, age sixty-eight, becomes the first pedestrian to be killed by an automobile. The car, driven by Arthur Smith, hits Mr. Bliss near the corner of 74th Street and Central Park West in New York City. **1916**: As punishment for killing three men, Mary, a circus elephant, is hanged in Erwin, Tennessee. The lynching is accomplished on the second try with a steel cable attached to a railroad derrick. Five thousand people watch. **1971**: Attica Prison Riot: twenty-eight prisoners and nine guards being held hostage are killed by gunfire during an assault on the prison by 1,500 guards, state troopers, and sheriff's deputies.   □ **SEPTEMBER 14, 1836**: Aaron Burr, third Vice President of the U.S., dies penniless in a hotel room in Staten Island, New York. **1901**: William McKinley, twenty-fourth President of the U.S., dies eight days after being shot by an assassin in Buffalo, New York. He is fifty-eight at the time of his death. His last words: "It is God's way. His will be done, not ours ... We are all going, we are all going, we are all going. Oh, dear." **1928**: Isadora Duncan is strangled when her scarf becomes tangled in the wheel of a Bugatti in Nice, France.   □ **SEPTEMBER 15, 1963**: Four young girls die at the 16th Street Baptist Church in Birmingham, Alabama, when a bomb explodes during Sunday services.   □ **SEPTEMBER 16, 1857**: The Mountain Meadow Massacre: Indians, led by Mormons, kill 120 men, women, and children in a wagon train crossing through Utah.   □ **SEPTEMBER 17, 1876**: The James Gang, during a raid on the First National Bank in Northfield, Minnesota, loses two of its eight members to bullet wounds. Within a few days, other members of the gang are wounded and killed by pursuing posses, making the Northfield raid the last major action of this outlaw group. **1908**: Thomas Selfridge, a lieutenant in the U.S. Signal Corps, becomes the first person to die in an airplane crash when a plane piloted by Orville Wright with Selfridge as an observer crashes in Fort Meyer, Florida. Wright is injured.   □ **SEPTEMBER 18, 1970**: After overdosing on sleeping pills, Jimi Hendrix, musician, suffocates on his own vomit and dies at the age of twenty-eight in London, England. □ **SEPTEMBER 19, 1881**: James Garfield twentieth President of the U.S., dies at the age of forty-nine in Elberon, New Jersey. The cause of death is blood poisoning caused by a gunshot wound received in an assassination attempt eighty days before at the Baltimore and Potomac Railway Depot, in Washington, D.C. □ **SEPTEMBER 20, 1973**: Jim Croce, composer and musician, dies at the age of thirty in a plane crash near the Natchitoches Municipal Airport in Louisiana. □ **SEPTEMBER 21, 1904**: Chief Joseph of the Nez Perce, dies in exile on a reservation in Colville, Washington. □ **SEPTEMBER 22, 1776**: Nathan Hale is hanged. □ **SEPTEM-BER 23, 1939**: Sigmund Freud, father of psychiatry, dies. □ **SEPTEMBER 24, 1904**: A railroad wreck in New Market, Tennessee, kills fifty-six. □ **SEPTEMBER 25, 1891**: A bomb explosion in Newark, New Jersey, kills eleven people.   □ **SEPTEMBER 26, 1945**: Bela Bartok, Hungarian composer, dies in New York City.   □ **SEPTEMBER 27, 1915**: A gasoline tank explodes in Ardmore, Oklahoma, killing forty-seven people.   □ **SEPTEMBER 28, 1970**: Gamal Abdel Nasser, age fifty-two, President of Egypt, dies from a heart attack in Cairo. □ **SEPTEMBER 29, 48 B.C.**: Pompey the Great is murdered in Egypt. □ **SEPTEMBER 30, 1630**:   John Billington becomes the first person to be executed in America. He is hanged for the crime of murder, having shot and killed an antagonist during an argument. **1955**: James Dean, actor, dies at age twenty-four near Paso Robles, California. He is driving more than eighty miles per hour in a silver Porsche Spyder when he collides with another automobile at the intersection of Route 466 and Route 41. While the driver of the other car receives only minor injuries and a passenger in the Porsche is also injured, the force of the crash almost severs Dean's head from his body.

OCTOBER

□ **OCTOBER 1, 1909**:   During a violent labor demonstration, a bomb explodes in the Los Angeles Times Building and kills twenty people. □ **OCTOBER 2, 322 B.C.**:   Aristotle dies of indigestion. **1970**: Thirteen members of the Wichita State University football team and their coach die in a plane crash in the mountains of Colorado, on their way to a game with Utah State. □ **OCTOBER 3, 1226**: Saint Francis of Assisi dies. □ **OCTOBER 4, 1930**: The British Airship *R-101* crashes in France, killing forty-seven people aboard, including the Secretary of State for Air and the Director of Civil Aviation. The disaster doomed furthur development of the airship in Great Britain. **1970**: In Hollywood, Janis Joplin, singer, dies at age twenty-seven of an apparent overdose of heroin.   □ **OCTOBER 5, 1892**: The Dalton Gang is almost destroyed during a bank raid in Coffeyville, Kansas; four gang members and four town residents are killed.   □ **OCTOBER 6, 1981**: Anwar Sadat, President of Egypt, dies from bullet wounds fired by an assassin. Sadat was attending a military review in Cairo at the time of his death. □ **OCTOBER 7, 1849**: Edgar Allen Poe, writer, dies. In a poem, he had described death as ". . . the play is the tragedy, 'Man,'/ And its hero, the Conqueror Worm." Dying, his last words are: "Lord help my poor soul." Although popularily attributed to alcohol abuse, his death is most likely from a brain tumor or diabetic coma. □ **OCTOBER 8, 1869**:   Franklin Pierce, fourteenth President of the U.S., dies of stomach inflammation in Concord, New Hampshire, at the age of sixty-four years. **1871**: The Great Chicago Fire starts. The death toll of 250 does not include seven men shot to death the next day as they attempt to start new fires (apparently to create looting opportunities). One other person is stoned to death by a mob. **1871**: The Great Pestigo Fire, a huge forest fire covering six counties in Wisconsin, kills 1,182 people. Due to the catastrophe in Chicago, this fire is virtually ignored by the press. **1967**: Che Guevara, Cuban revolutionary leader, dies from gunshot wounds sustained after his capture by army forces in Bolivia. He is thirty-nine.   □ **OCTOBER 9, 1963**: A massive landslide in Belluno, Italy, kills 2,000 people.   □ **OCTOBER 10, 1947**: The first shipload of American dead from World War II's Pacific theater arrives in San Francisco, California. The ship is carrying 3,028 coffins.   □ **OCTOBER 11, 1737**: A violent earthquake hits Calcutta, India, killing 30,000.   □ **OCTOBER 12, 1870**: Robert E. Lee, military leader of the Confederate Army, dies in Lexington, Virginia. A recent flood had washed away a shipment of coffins, so a search is undertaken to find one in which to bury the General. The only one found is too short for Lee's body; in order to fit him in, he has to be buried with his shoes off.   □ **OCTOBER 13, 1894**: During a drunken riot in Maltby — an Hungarian community near Wilkes-Barre, Pennsylvania — a boy is shot and killed.   □ **OCTOBER 14, 1977**: Bing Crosby dies. His last words: "That was a great game of golf, fellers."   □ **OCTOBER 15, 1917**: Mata Hari, exotic dancer, is executed by a firing squad in Vincennes, France, after being convicted of spying. Although there are twelve members of the firing squad plus an officer shooting at her, an autopsy indicates that only four bullets hit her body. **1946**: Hermann Goering, convicted Nazi war criminal, poisons himself in Nuremburg Prison in Germany — two hours before his scheduled hanging. □ **OCTOBER 16, 1793**:   Marie Antoinette, deposed Queen of France, loses her head to the guillotine in Paris.   □ **OCTOBER 17, 1814**: A rupture in a tank in a brewery in London sends 3,500 barrels of beer flooding through a densely populated area of the city. Nine people are killed.   □ **OCTOBER 18, 1931**: Thomas Alva Edison, inventor, dies in West Orange, New Jersey, at the age of eighty-three, after being in a coma for five days.   □ **OCTOBER 19, 1881**: Pilot the dog, becomes the American Champion fighting dog by killing Crib, his opponent, after one hour and twenty-five minutes of combat, near Louisville, Kentucky.   □ **OCTOBER 20, 1964**: Herbert Hoover, thirtieth President of the U.S., dies at his home in New York City at the age of ninety years. The cause of death is listed as bleeding from the upper gastrointestinal tract and a strained vascular system. He is buried at West Branch, Iowa.   □ **OCTOBER 21, 1805**: Admiral Horatio Nelson dies after being wounded during a naval battle. His last words: "Thank God I have done my duty."   □ **OCTOBER 22, 1934**: Charles Arthur "Pretty Boy" Floyd, Public Enemy Number One, dies in a cornfield near East Liverpool, Ohio, after being shot eight times by FBI agents.

He is thirty-three years old. ☐ **OCTOBER 23, 1950**: Al Jolson, comedian, dies while playing cards at the St. Francis Hotel in San Francisco, California. Cause of death: heart attack. ☐ **OCTOBER 24, 1871**: During a vicious riot in the Chinatown section of Los Angeles, California, a mob killed about twenty-five Chinese area residents. No one is ever tried for these crimes, but public pressure eventually forces city officials to change the name of the main street in the Chinese section from Nigger Alley to Los Angeles Street. **1931**: The George Washington Bridge over the Hudson River in New York City opens to traffic after four years of construction and twelve deaths. ☐ **OCTOBER 25, 1957**: Albert Anastasia, Lord High Executioner of Murder, Inc., is murdered by two unknown gunmen in the barber shop of the Park Sheraton Hotel in New York City. ☐ **OCTOBER 26, 1881**: Three die in the gunfight at the O.K. Corral. ☐ **OCTOBER 27, 1925**: Twenty-five people die in a railroad wreck in Victoria, Mississippi. ☐ **OCTOBER 28, 1893**: Carter Harrison, the mayor of Chicago, Illinois, is assassinated. ☐ **OCTOBER 29, 1971**: Duane Allman, musician, dies in a hospital in Macon, Georgia, after hours of surgery following a crash on his motorcycle. He is twenty-five years old. ☐ **OCTOBER 30, 1912**: James Schoolcraft Sherman, the twenty-seventh Vice President of the U.S., dies in Utica, New York, of uremic poisoning only a few days before the election for his and Taft's second term. No replacement was offered by the party, and 3,484,980 people cast their votes for a dead man on election day. ☐ **OCTOBER 31, 1880**: During the height of Denver's Chinese riots, an angry mob lynchs a Chinese man from a lamppost. Many other Chinese are attacked and killed in other cities during a wave of anti-Chinese sentiment. During this period, Henry Ward Beecher said, "We have clubbed them, stoned them, burned their houses and murdered some of them; yet they refuse to be converted. I do not know any way, except to blow them up with nitroglycerin, if we are ever to get them to Heaven."

NOVEMBER

☐ **NOVEMBER 1, 1955**: A bomb planted on a United Airlines flight explodes and the plane crashes in Longmont, Colorado. Forty-four people die. The bomb was placed on board to kill a passenger in order for her son to collect insurance. ☐ **NOVEMBER 2, 1950**: George Bernard Shaw, playwright, dies in England at age ninety-four. He was suffering from a kidney infection and was weak from a fall suffered on September 11. The broken bone that resulted from the fall prompted him to say, "When one is very old your legs give in before your head does." **1965**: Norman Morrison, Quaker, dies from burns suffered when he set himself afire outside the Pentagon office window of Defense Secretary Robert McNamara. Morrison was protesting the U.S. involvement in Vietnam. ☐ **NOVEMBER 3, 1963**: In New York City, eleven of a car's twelve occupants die after driving off a dead end street and into the Harlem River. ☐ **NOVEMBER 4, 1856**: A political riot between Democrats and the Know-Nothing Party leaves eight people dead in Baltimore, Maryland.

□ **NOVEMBER 5, 1979**:   Al Capp, cartoonist, dies from emphysema.
□ **NOVEMBER 6, 1873**:   After they are captured on board a ship carrying arms to Cuban rebels, thirty Americans are shot to death by Spanish soldiers.
□ **NOVEMBER 7, 1962**:   Eleanor Roosevelt, the "First Lady of the World," dies at the age of seventy-eight in her home in New York City, from the effects of a lung infection and anemia. **1967**: John Nance Garner, thirty-second Vice President of the U.S., dies in Uvalde, Texas.   □ **NOVEMBER 8, 1887**: After drinking a glass of whiskey, "Doc" Holliday, dentist, dies at the age of thirty-five in a sanitorium in Glenwood Springs, Colorado. His last words: "I'll be damned!" He had been suffering from tuberculosis for many years.
□ **NOVEMBER 9, 1974**:   Naptha, leaking from a collision between two ships in Japan's Tokyo Bay, catches fire. Thirty-three die.   □ **NOVEMBER 10, 1796**: Catherine the Great of Russia dies from apoplexy at the age of sixty-seven. **1865**: Henry Wirz, who was in charge of Andersonville prison in Georgia, becomes the only war criminal from the Civil War to be executed. When sentenced, he said, "I'm damned if the Yankee eagle hasn't turned out to be what I expected, a damned turkey buzzard." **1898**: White citizens in Wilmington, North Carolina massacre 100 blacks.   □ **NOVEMBER 11, 1938**: Typhoid Mary dies while under detention on North Brother Island on the East River in New York City. Seven separate typhoid epidemics were linked to her. Estimates of deaths resulting from the disease range from a few hundred to more than 1,000. **1945**: Jerome Kern, composer, dies in a hospital in New York City. He had been unconscious for several days after collapsing on the corner of 57th Street and Park Avenue. Oscar Hammerstein II tried in vain to revive his friend by singing "Ol' Man River" in his ear.   □ **NOVEMBER 12, 1872**: The Great Boston Fire, which started November 9, is finally put out, leaving eighty acres destroyed and thirty-five people dead.   □ **NOVEMBER 13, 1965**: The cruise ship, *Yarmouth Castle*, en route to the Bahamas, catches fire and sinks, killing ninety passengers. Most of the deaths result from inadequate safety and lifesaving equipment.   □ **NOVEMBER 14, 1970**: Forty-three members of the Marshall University football team are killed in a charter plane crash in Kenova, West Virginia.   □ **NOVEMBER 15, 1959**: The Clutter family is murdered *In Cold Blood* near Holcomb, Kansas. Richard Hickock and Perry Smith are convicted and hanged for the crime in April, 1965.   □ **NOVEMBER 16, 1959**: Forty-two people aboard a National Airlines plane die when it crashes into the Gulf of Mexico near New Orleans, Louisiana.   □ **NOVEMBER 17, 1949**: While on a training flight, two B-29 bombers collide 27,000 feet above Stockton, California, killing eighteen of the twenty-one crewmen. **1953**: During a mass parachute drop at Fort Bragg, North Carolina, a C-119 crashes, killing fifteen men. Nine of the dead were paratroopers who were hit by the plane on its way down. **1965**: Henry A. Wallace, thirty-third Vice President of the U.S., dies in Danbury, Connecticut.   □ **NOVEMBER 18, 1886**: Chester A. Arthur, twenty-first President of the U.S., dies in New York City, at the age of fifty-seven. The cause of death: a cerebral hemorrhage. **1978**: Jim Jones, religious leader of the People's Temple, dies from a self-inflicted bullet wound in Jonestown,

Guyana. Along with Jones, 910 followers of his philosophy die, most from drinking Kool-Aid mixed with cyanide. In addition, Representative Leo Ryan from California and four members of his staff — all of whom were investigating the People's Temple — are shot to death near the temple site. □ **NOVEMBER 19, 1828:** Franz Schubert, composer, dies from the effects of typhoid fever. He is buried next to Beethoven. **1850:** Richard Mentor Johnson, ninth Vice President of the U.S., dies of a stroke in Frankfort, Kentucky. A regional newspaper had reported previously that he had been suffering from "an attack of dementia."   □ **NOVEMBER 20, 1975:** Francisco Franco, dictator of Spain, dies at the age of eighty-two in La Paz Hospital in Madrid. □ **NOVEMBER 21, 1899:**   Garret Augustus Hobart, twenty-fourth Vice President of the U.S., dies from heart problems in Paterson, New Jersey. **1945:** Robert Benchley, actor, humorist, critic, dies at age fifty-six in New York City. His last words are written on the title page of a book entitled *Am I Thinking?*, which he had been reading: "No. And supposing you were?" **1718:** After an intense struggle in which he is shot five times and cut twenty-five times by a cutlass, Edward "Blackbeard the Pirate" Teach dies near Ocracoke Island, North Carolina. The fight ends when someone hits him from behind with a sword, severing his head.   □ **NOVEMBER 22, 1875:** Henry Wilson, eighteenth Vice President of the U.S., dies in Washington, D.C., twelve days after suffering an apoplectic stroke during a bath. One of the treatments used was an injection of whiskey into his shoulder. **1963:** John F. Kennedy, thirty-fifth President of the U.S., is assassinated in Dallas, Texas. He was forty-six years old. His last words: "My God, I've been hit." **1963:** Aldous Huxley, writer, dies of throat cancer in Santa Barbara, California. With his doctor's consent, he dies under the influence of LSD.   □ **NOVEMBER 23, 1814:** On his way home in a carriage from the Capitol in Washington, D.C., Elbridge Gerry, the fifth Vice President of the U.S., dies of a hemorrhage.   □ **NOVEMBER 24, 1983:** At a San Francisco nightclub, a man is crushed to death between the ceiling and a prop piano that was engineered to rise from the stage to the ceiling. Apparently, he and a girl friend had been making love on top of the piano when the switch controlling its movement was accidentally triggered.   □ **NOVEMBER 25, 2348 B.C.:** The Great Flood, according to some biblical scholars. Everyone not on the Ark with Noah perishes. **1885:** Thomas Andrews Hendricks, twenty-first Vice President of the U.S., dies in Indianapolis, Indiana, after a prolonged illness. **1944:** A German V-2 rocket lands on a Woolworth's store on New Cross Road in Deptford, London, England, killing 160 shoppers and store personnel. □ **NOVEMBER 26, 1933:**   During a violent hailstorm in South Africa, two children, 2,000 sheep, and 250 cattle are killed.   □ **NOVEMBER 27, 1934:** George "Baby Face" Nelson, Public Enemy, dies at the age of twenty-six — after receiving seventeen bullet wounds from FBI agents during a gun battle in a ditch near Barrington, Illinois.   □ **NOVEMBER 28, 1893:** A piano tuner is stoned to death by a mob near Winchester, Illinois. Details of this incident are not available.   □ **NOVEMBER 29, 1872:** A few days after his defeat by Ulysses Grant in the Presidential race, Horace Greeley dies of exhaustion in

Pleasantville, New York.   □ **NOVEMBER 30, 1889**: The Tribune Building in Minneapolis, Minnesota, burns, killing ten people.

DECEMBER

□ **DECEMBER 1, 1958**:   A fire in Our Lady of the Angels parochial school in Chicago, Illinois, leaves ninety-two children and three nuns dead. □ **DECEMBER 2, 1859**:   John Brown is hanged in Charleston, West Virginia. His last words: "Don't keep me waiting any longer than necessary." □ **DECEMBER 3, 1910**:   Mary Baker Eddy, founder of the Christian Science Church, dies while battling a cold. Believing that no illness could hurt her, she attributes the cold to evil forces.   □ **DECEMBER 4, 1969**: Fred Hampton and Mark Clark, Black Panther Party leaders, die from gunshot wounds during a police raid in Chicago, Illinois.   □ **DECEMBER 5, 1791**: Wolfgang Amadeus Mozart, composer, dies at the age of thirty-five, after feeling sick for weeks. The day before, he had remarked, "I have the flavor of death on my tongue. I taste death." **1876**: The Brooklyn Theater in New York City burns, killing 289 people. (A survey done at that time reported that one out of every four theaters burned within four years of being built.)   □ **DECEMBER 6, 1917**: A munition ship explodes in the harbor at Halifax, Nova Scotia, killing 1,226 people and burning one-third of the city.   □ **DECEMBER 7, 1817**: Captain Bligh, famous shipboard tyrant, dies.   □ **DECEMBER 8, 1930**: In Bombay, India, thirty people die from eating soup made from a poisonous lizard. **1931**: "Legs" Diamond is murdered in Albany, New York, the day after he was acquitted on a kidnapping charge.   □ **DECEMBER 9, 1926**: Francisco Mine No. 2, in Francisco, Indiana, explodes from an accumulation of gas, killing thirty-seven miners.   □ **DECEMBER 10, 1967**: Otis Redding, composer and singer, dies at age twenty-six in a plane crash in Lake Monona, near Madison, Wisconsin.   □ **DECEMBER 11, 1964**: Sam Cooke, singer, dies at age twenty-nine, in a motel room in Los Angeles, California, after being shot three times by a woman who described him as an assailant.   □ **DECEMBER 12, 1976**: Jack Cassidy, actor, dies at age forty-nine in Los Angeles, California. Burned beyond recognition in a fire that destroyed his apartment, he was identified by his dental records.   □ **DECEMBER 13, 1922**: A train wreck in Humble, Texas kills twenty-two people.   □ **DECEMBER 14, 1799**: George Washington dies after being bled by physicians who are trying to cure his laryngitis. He is sixty-seven years old. His last words: "It is well."   □ **DECEMBER 15, 1890**: Sitting Bull, Sioux Chief, is assassinated by Indian police in South Dakota.   □ **DECEMBER 16, 1916**: Grigori Rasputin, mystic and advisor to the Russian royal family, dies at the hands of his enemies. He is poisoned with potassium cyanide, shot once in the back and twice in the front, beaten, and shoved through a hole in the ice of a river in St. Petersburg.   □ **DECEMBER 17, 63 A.D.**: Lazarus dies for the second time. **1983**: A fire in a discotheque in Madrid, Spain, kills seventy-eight. □ **DECEMBER 18, 1948**:   Two buses collide in Utah, killing thirteen people. **1966**: Two buses collide near Qum, Iran, killing twenty-five people. **1970**: A bus near Rawalpindi, India drives off a bridge. Twenty-six people drown. □ **DECEMBER 19, 1948**: New York City receives 19.6 inches of snow, causing five deaths. □ **DECEMBER 20, 1968**: John Steinbeck, author, dies. □ **DECEMBER 21, 1945**: General George S. Patton, Jr., commander of the 15th U.S. Army, dies from the injuries he received in an automobile accident in Mannheim, Germany, on December 9. **1967**: Louis Washkansky, age fifty-five, dies of double pneumonia in a hospital in Capetown, South Africa. He had lived for eighteen days with the first transplanted heart. □ **DECEMBER 22, 1972**: An earthquake in Managua, Nicaragua, kills 5,000 people. **1977**: A grain dust explosion in Westwego, Louisiana, kills thirty-five workers. □ **DECEMBER 23, 1862**: In the largest execution in U.S. history, thirty-eight Sioux Indians are hanged in Mankato, Minnesota. □ **DECEMBER 24, 1872**: A railroad bridge collapses under a train in Corry, Pennsylvania; twenty people are killed. □ **DECEMBER 25, 1946**: W. C. Fields, comedian and juggler, dies from the effects of excessive drinking at his home in Hollywood, California. □ **DECEMBER 26, 1972**: Harry Truman, thirty-third President of the U.S., dies in Independence, Missouri, at the age of eighty-eight. Cause of death: collapse of his cardiovascular system, along with other system failures. His last words: "I'm a broken machine, but I'm ready." □ **DECEMBER 27, 1969**: Reports from Zambia recount the deaths of nine people on the Namwala River. Their boats were overturned by rampaging hippopotamuses. □ **DECEMBER 28, 1908**: An earthquake in Messina, Sicily, kills 85,000 people □ **DECEMBER 29, 1170**: Thomas Becket is murdered. **1975**: A bomb explodes in the main passenger terminal at La Guardia airport in New York City, killing eleven people. □ **DECEMBER 30, 1903**: The Iroquois Theater burns in Chicago, Illinois, during a performance by Eddie Foy; 602 people are killed. □ **DECEMBER 31, 1864**: George Mifflin Dallas, eleventh Vice President of the U.S., dies in Philadelphia, Pennsylvania. **1972**: Roberto Clemente, baseball player, dies at the age of thirty-eight in a plane crash near San Juan, Puerto Rico. He was accompanying supplies being flown to victims of an earthquake in Nicaragua.

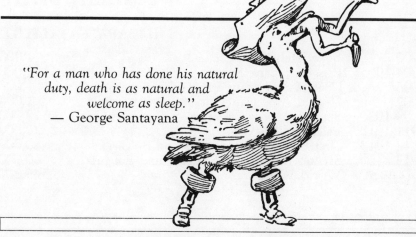

"For a man who has done his natural
duty, death is as natural and
welcome as sleep."
— George Santayana

It's all a world where bugs and
emperors
Go singularly back to the same dust."
— Edwin Arlington Robinson

APPENDIX

TWENTIETH CENTURY WAR DEATHS
An Incomplete Roll Of Modern Human Strife

		MILITARY FATALITIES
1900	Boxer Rebellion, China	1,000
1904-1905	Russian-Japanese War	130,000
1906	Central American War, Cuban uprising	1,000
1907	Central American War, Honduran revolt	1,000
1909-1910	Spanish-Moroccan War	10,000
1911-1912	Italo-Turkish War	20,000
1912-1913	First Balkan War, Turkey and Bulgaria	80,000
1913	Second Balkan War, Turkey and Bulgaria	60,000
1914-1918	World War I	8,545,800

FATALITIES

1916	U.S. vs. Pancho Villa	420
1918-1921	Russian Civil War	50,000
1919	Hungarian Allies War	10,000
1921	Greek-Turkish War	50,000
1921-1926	Riffian War, France and Spain	30,000
1925-1927	Druze War, Syria	5,000
1931-1933	Manchurian War, Japan and China	60,000
1932-1935	Chaco War, Paraguay and Bolivia	130,000
1935-1936	Italian-Ethiopian War	20,000
1936-1939	Spanish Civil War	611,000
1937-1941	Sino-Japanese War	1,000,000
1939	Russian-Japanese War	19,000
1939-1940	Russian-Finnish War	90,000
1939-1945	World War II	15,843,000
1945-1946	Indonesian Independence	1,400
1945-1954	Indo-Chinese War, France and Vietminh	100,000
1947	India-Pakistan War	200,000
1947-1949	First Kashmir War, India and Pakistan	1,500
1948-1949	Israeli Independence War	8,000
1950-1953	Korean War	1,893,100
1952-1955	Kenyan War, Kenya and Great Britain	800
1954-1962	Algerian War, Revolt against French	15,000
1956	Hungarian Uprising	30,000
1956	Sinai War, Israel and U.A.R.	3,230
1956-1959	Tibetan Invasion, U.S.S.R. and Tibet	40,000
1956-1959	Cuban Revolution	50,000
1961-1973	Vietnam War	546,000
1962	Sino-Indian War	1,000
1965	Second Kashmir War, Pakistan and India	7,000
1967	Six Day War, Israel and Arab States	21,000
1967-1970	Biafran Uprising, Nigeria	1,000,000
1969-1978	Rhodesian Civil War	6,000
1969	Football War, Honduras and Salvador	2,000
1978-1979	Uganda-Tanzanian War	10,000
1979-	Afghanistan Invasion, U.S.S.R.	200,000
1980-	Iran-Iraq War	200,000
1982	Falkland Islands War, Argentina and G.B.	1,250

The Grand Total, and growing: 31,104,000

DEATH RATES FOR

STATE RANKINGS

	Death Rate	Heart Deaths	Cancer Deaths	Stroke Deaths	Pulmonary Deaths	Accident Deaths	Suicide Deaths
Alabama	18	32	24	9	11	36	32
Alaska	50	50	50	50	1	50	3
Arizona	38	42	38	43	12	1	4
Arkansas	5	11	10	1	13	28	29
California	40	39	33	31	30	26	10
Colorado	47	46	46	45	29	9	5
Connecticut	23	23	8	36	45	34	48
Delaware	28	19	17	44	36	29	25
Florida	1	5	1	2	21	3	7
Georgia	34	39	42	16	14	41	19
Hawaii	49	49	48	49	46	49	31
Idaho	44	43	44	40	7	27	15
Illinois	20	9	18	28	38	37	46
Indiana	25	24	23	14	37	30	42
Iowa	14	12	12	6	31	11	37
Kansas	15	16	27	12	16	15	39
Kentucky	16	14	21	11	24	10	17
Louisianna	27	30	36	23	10	47	24
Maine	11	13	4	13	35	2	21
Maryland	37	31	19	42	43	45	40
Massachusetts	8	8	5	27	44	23	49
Michigan	36	27	30	39	40	35	30
Minnesota	33	29	32	22	33	40	41
Mississippi	9	25	28	4	6	44	47
Missouri	3	7	9	10	17	18	26
Montana	29	34	37	29	3	5	11
Nebraska	17	20	15	5	26	17	43
Nevada	43	44	41	46	5	8	1
New Hampshire	30	28	14	37	48	16	38
New Jersey	12	6	7	32	49	31	50
New Mexico	45	48	45	47	4	12	2
New York	7	2	6	33	50	32	45
North Carolina	32	33	35	17	20	42	33
North Dakota	26	22	39	19	22	33	36
Ohio	19	15	11	26	41	24	27
Oklahoma	13	17	22	7	9	21	16
Oregon	31	36	29	25	25	7	9
Pennsylvania	2	1	3	18	42	19	35
Rhode Island	6	4	2	24	47	13	34
South Carolina	35	37	40	20	18	46	44
South Dakota	10	10	26	8	8	25	18
Tennessee	22	26	25	3	23	22	23
Texas	42	41	43	34	19	43	22
Utah	48	47	49	48	34	48	14
Vermont	21	21	13	38	28	4	8
Virginia	39	35	31	30	32	39	12
Washington	41	40	34	35	27	14	13
West Virginia	4	3	16	15	15	6	20
Wisconsin	24	18	20	21	39	38	28
Wyoming	46	45	47	41	2	20	6

THE STATES - 1980

STATE RANKINGS

Homicide Deaths	Population Density	Median Age	Median Income	Divorce Rate	Physician Ratio	Birth Rate	
13	27	31	44	11	48	27	Alabama
1	50	49	1	2	16	2	Alaska
22	41	30	29	6	36	11	Arizona
23	36	9	50	12	49	28	Arkansas
10	14	20	12	21	13	18	California
28	39	38	11	16	11	16	Colorado
33	4	4	3	37	1	50	Connecticut
31	7	25	17	43	35	33	Delaware
6	11	1	36	7	38	45	Florida
7	23	39	38	17	43	19	Georgia
40	15	40	2	32	8	10	Hawaii
43	21	45	40	9	24	4	Idaho
21	10	21	7	34	20	21	Illinois
25	13	33	18	8	39	30	Indiana
44	33	19	22	41	21	26	Iowa
29	38	17	26	20	31	17	Kansas
16	24	34	46	33	33	29	Kentucky
3	22	47	47	38	45	6	Louisana
48	37	11	48	23	34	41	Maine
14	5	12	4	40	15	13	Maryland
37	3	7	13	49	3	49	Massachusetts
20	12	37	8	29	18	35	Michigan
45	34	32	14	45	7	23	Minnesota
4	32	44	49	24	50	9	Mississippi
17	28	8	32	22	28	31	Missouri
36	48	35	31	18	14	13	Montana
49	42	26	30	39	9	14	Nebraska
5	47	14	9	1	40	20	Nevada
47	20	18	25	19	23	39	New Hampshire
26	1	2	5	44	6	47	New Jersey
8	44	46	41	4	37	5	New Mexico
9	6	5	20	47	2	44	New York
19	17	27	42	31	46	42	North Carolina
50	45	41	33	48	30	12	North Dakota
27	9	22	16	25	25	34	Ohio
12	35	15	34	5	41	15	Oklahoma
34	40	13	24	14	4	25	Oregon
30	8	3	21	50	19	46	Pennsylvania
38	2	6	27	30	22	48	Rhode Island
11	19	43	39	36	47	22	South Carolina
42	46	36	45	42	29	8	South Dakota
15	18	16	47	15	26	37	Tennessee
2	31	42	28	13	42	7	Texas
39	43	50	23	26	10	1	Utah
46	30	29	37	28	17	36	Vermont
24	16	24	19	35	27	40	Virginia
35	29	23	10	10	5	24	Washington
32	26	10	43	27	44	38	West Virginia
41	25	28	15	46	12	32	Wisconsin
18	49	48	6	3	32	3	Wyoming

U.S.A. DEATHS AND DEATH RATES — 1980

CAUSES OF DEATH	RATE (per 100,000)	FATALITIES
Cardiovascular Diseases	**436.4**	**988,500**
— Heart Disease	332.4	761,100
— Stroke	75.1	170,200
— Others	28.9	57,200
Malignancies (Cancer)	183.9	416,500
Accidents — Adverse Effects	**46.7**	**105,700**
— Motor Vehicle	23.5	53,200
— Others	23.2	52,500
Chronic Pulmonary Obstruction	24.7	56,100
Pneumonia and Influenza	24.1	54,600
Diabetes Mellitus	15.4	34,900
Chronic Liver Diseases	13.5	30,600
Perinatal Condictions	10.1	22,900
Suicide	11.9	26,900
Homicide — Legal Intervention	10.7	24,300
Nephritis — Nephrosis	7.4	16,800
Congenital Anomalies	6.2	13,900
Septicemia	4.2	9,400
Ulcers	2.7	6,100
Benign Neoplasms	2.7	6,200
Hernia — Intestinal Obstruction	2.4	5,400
Other Diseases	2.2	5,100
Anemias	1.4	3,200
Cholethiasis	1.5	3,300
Kidney Infections	1.2	2,700
Nutritional Deficiencies	1.0	2,400
Tuberculosis	.9	2,000
Meningitus	.6	1,400
Hyperplasia of Prostate	.3	800
Bronchitis — Bronchiolitis	.3	600
Viral Hepatitis	.4	800
Ill Defined Conditions	12.7	28,800
All Other Causes	53.0	120,000
All Causes	**878.3**	**1,989,800**

"When death comes, he respects neither age nor merit. He sweeps from this earthly existence the sick and the strong, the rich and the poor, and should teach us to live to be prepared for death."
— Andrew Jackson

INDEX

ABBANDANDO, FRANK 187
ABORTIONS 116, 126–127
ACCIDENTS 13, 15, 18, 56–69, 88, 214
ACCIDENTS, TRANSPORTATION 70–87
ADAMS, JOHN QUINCY 16, 188, 197
ADDICTIVE DRUGS 103
ADENAUER, KONRAD 192
AERIAL BOMBING 141, 142, 151, 153
AGRICULTURE 64
AGUE 23
AIR FORCE 79, 80, 138, 139
AIRPLANES 81, 82, 83–84, 85, 87
ALBERT I 187
ALCOHOL 77, 80, 101, 104, 111, 114
ALCOHOL ABUSE 100
ALCOHOL POISONING 106
ALCOHOLICS 35, 92
ALEXANDER II 174
ALEXANDER THE GREAT 23, 196
ALLMAN, DUANE 205
AMEBIASIS 24
AMMUNITION EXPENDITURE 140, 141, 142
AMPUTATIONS 51
ANAPHYLACTIC SHOCK 178
ANASTASIA, ALBERT 205
ANEMIA 107, 214
ANESTHETICS 51
ANEURYSM 33
ANGINA 30, 31
ANIMAL FATALITIES 163
ANIMAL KILLERS 178–183
ANIMALS 44
ANTS 178
ANTHRAX 148, 149
ANTHROPOPHAGY 127

ANTI-AIRCRAFT WEAPONS 142
ANTI-SOCIAL BEHAVIOR 88, 128
ANTIBIOTICS 42, 46
ANTISEPTIC SURGERY 51
ANTOINETTE, MARIE 124, 204
ARBUCKLE, FATTY 196
ARCHBISHOP OF CANTERBURY 184
ARISTOTLE 203
ARMY 79, 80, 135, 138, 139
ARMY AIR CORPS 138
ARMY HOSPITALS 136
ARMY TACTICS 140
ARNOLD, BENEDICT 196
ARSON 112
ARTERIES 28, 30, 33
ARTERIOSCLEROSIS 28, 30, 33
ARTHUR, CHESTER A. 206
ARTILLERY 141
ASBESTOSIS 66
ASIAN FLU 46
ASSASSINATIONS 16, 108, 115–116, 133
ASTOR, JOHN JACOB 190
ATHLETIC EVENTS 164
ATOMIC BOMB 152, 153, 154
ATOMIC BOMBING OF AMERICANS 153
AUDUBON, JOHN JAMES 186
AUSTIN, JANE 198
AUTO ACCIDENTS 33, 38, 54, 60, 77, 87
AUTOEROTIC ASPHYXIA 107
AUTOPSIES 13–14, 52, 53, 120, 143
AVALANCHES 168–169
AVERAGE LIFETIME 12
AVIATION ACCIDENTS 18, 83

BABY KILLING   125
BACTERIA   45
BARKER, MA   185
BARKLEY, ALBEN W.   193
BARRACUDAS   180
BARRETT, MICHAEL   194
BARRYMORE, JOHN   194
BARTOK, BELA   203
BASSETT, CHARLES   188
BATS   44
BATTLEFIELD TACTICS   140
BEARS   180
BEATINGS   112, 121
BECKET, THOMAS   209
BEECHER, HENRY WARD   205
BEES   177
BEETHOVEN   190
BEHAN, BRENDAN   102
BEHEADINGS   117
BELL RINGERS   164
BELUSHI, JOHN   102
BENCHLEY, ROBERT   207
BETHEA, RAINEY   117
BICYCLES   75, 76
BIDDLE, JOHN   130
"THE BIG BOPPER"   186
BILHARZIASIS   24
BILLINGTON, JOHN   203
BILLY THE KID   198
BIOLOGICAL WEAPONS   148
BIORHYTHMS   17–18
BIRTH   41, 42, 50, 53
BIRTH RATE   10, 213
BLACK BEARS   180
"BLACK HUNDREDS"   156
BLACK LUNG DISEASE   66
BLACK PLAGUE   45, 155
"BLACK SEPTEMBER" TERRORISTS
     202
BLACK WIDOW SPIDERS   178
"BLACKBEARD THE PIRATE"   207
BLADDER   40
BLAKE, WILLIAM   200
BLISS, HENRY   202
BLOOD   30, 33, 55, 69
BLOOD VESSELS   22, 31, 32, 69
BLOOMFIELD, MICHAEL   102, 187
BLUNT OBJECTS   112
BOCCALINI, TRAJAN   130
BODY COSTS   137
BODY COUNTS   138
BOGART, HUMPHREY   185
BOLEYN, ANNE   123
BOMBING STATISTICS   141, 142
BONAPARTE, NAPOLEON   193
BONES   40, 87
BONNIE AND CLYDE   194
BOOTH, JOHN WILKES   191
BORDEN, LIZZIE   200
BOTTLED GAS   65

BOYD, WILLIAM   202
BRADY, "DIAMOND JIM"   191
BRAIN   9, 25, 31, 32, 33, 40, 69
BRAUTIGAN, RICHARD   89
BREAST CANCER   40
BRECKENRIDGE, JOHN CABELL   194
BRIDGES   68, 69
BRONCHITIS   214
BRONZE AGE   11
BROWN SPIDERS   178
BROWN, JOHN   208
BRUCE, LENNY   102, 200
BUBONIC PLAGUE   44, 45, 49
BUDDHISTS   159
BUILDING FAILURES   67
BURBANK, LUTHER   191
BUREN, MARTIN VAN   199
BURKE, WILLIAM   186
BURNING ALIVE   121
BURNING BODIES   176
BURNS   58, 62, 65
BURR, AARON   202
BURROUGHS, EDGAR RICE   189

CAESAR, JULIUS   23, 174, 189
"CALAMITY JANE"   200
CALDER, ALEXANDER   184
CALHOUN, JOHN C.   190
CAMPING   164
CAMUS, ALBERT   87, 184
CANCER   13, 24, 37–41, 56, 88, 212, 214
CANINE DISTEMPER   44
CANINES   179
CANNARY, MARTHA   200
CANNIBALISM   20, 25–26, 127–129
CAPITAL PUNISHMENT   118
CAPONE, ALPHONSE "SCARFACE"
     186
CAPP, AL   206
CAPTAIN BLIGH   208
CAR EXHAUST POISONING   101
CARDIAC ARREST   15
CARDIOVASCULAR DISEASE   28, 32,
     54, 55, 214
CARELESSNESS   53
CASANOVA   195
CASSIDY, JACK   208
CATHERINE THE GREAT   206
CATHOLICS   88, 157
CATS   178–179
CAUSE OF DEATH   36, 33, 49
CEMETERIES   52
CEREBRAL EMBOLISM   33
CEREBRAL HEMORRHAGE   33
CEREBRAL THROMBOSIS   31, 33
CEREBROVASCULAR DISEASE   31, 32
CEREBROVASCULAR OCCLUSION
     33
CERMAK, ANTON   115, 133, 189

CERVIX CANCER   40
CHADWICK, ROY   201
CHAFFEE, ROGER   186
CHANCES OF BEING MURDERED
   110
CHANG AND ENG   185
CHARLES I   124
CHARLES II   187
CHEESE WAR   154
CHEKHOV, ANTON   197
CHEMICAL WEAPONS   147, 149
CHEMICALS   37, 61, 147, 149
CHESSMAN, CARYL   193
CHICKAMAUGA, BATTLE OF   159
CHIEF JOSEPH   203
CHILD ABUSE   124
CHILDBIRTH   41, 42
CHILDREN   20, 21, 25, 38, 40, 76
CHINA   19, 20, 21
CHLORINE GAS   146
CHOKING   58
CHOLERA   149
CHOLESTEROL   28, 32
CHRISTIANS   88, 97, 98, 125, 157
CHRISTIE, AGATHA   185
CHRONIC HEALTH PROBLEMS   101,
   104
CHRONIC PULMONARY OBSTRUCTIONS
   33, 214
CHURCH TOWERS   163
CHURCHILL, WINSTON   186
CIRCULATORY SYSTEM   31, 69
CIRRHOSIS OF THE LIVER   101, 104
CIVIL EXECUTIONS   117
CIVILIAN WAR DEATHS   151
CLARK, MARK   208
CLEMENS, SAMUEL   192
CLEMENTE, ROBERTO   87, 209
CLEOPATRA   89, 201
CLEVELAND, GROVER   196
CLINTON, GEORGE   192
COAL SLAG   169
COAST GUARD   138
COBRAS   182
COCAINE   17, 103
COFFINS   52, 61
COLE, NAT KING   187
COLFAX, SCHUYLER   185
COLLINS, MICHAEL   201
COLON CANCER   40
COMA   9
COMBAT FATALITIES   108, 135, 138,
   210, 211
COMBUSTIBLE MATERIALS   61
COMMUNIST PURGES   156
CONE SHELLS   181
CONGENITAL ANOMALIES   214
CONGENITAL HEART DISEASE   31
CONSTRUCTION   64, 68
CONSUMPTION   106

CONTINENTS, DISASTERS ON   161
COOK, CAPTIAN JAMES   187
COOKE, SAM   208
COOLIDGE, CALVIN   184
COOPER, GARY   193
COPPERHEAD SNAKES   178
CORAL SNAKES   178
CORBETT, JAMES "GENTLEMAN JIM"
   187
CORONARY HEART DISEASE   28
CORONARY OCCULSION   30
CORONARY THROMBOSIS   30
CORONERS   14, 15, 100
CORPSES   51, 52
COST PER BATTLE FATALITY   137
COWPOX   44
CRANE, HART   192
CRANE, STEPHEN   195
CRAWFORD, JOAN   193
CRIMINAL EXECUTIONS   117
CRIMINAL NEGLIGENCE   108
CROCE, JIM   87, 203
CROCODILE MASSACRE   180
CROMWELL, THOMAS   199
CROSBY, BING   204
CROWDS   132
CRUSADES   97, 155, 157
CURTIS, CHARLES   187
CUSTER, GEORGE ARMSTRONG   18,
   106
CVD   26, 27, 28, 29, 30, 32
CYCLES   17
CYPRUS   158

D'ASCOLI, CECCO   131
DALLAS, GEORGE MIFFLIN   209
"DANCE OF DEATH"   201
DARWIN, CHARLES   192
DAVIES, RODGER P.   116
DAWES, CHARLES G.   192
DDT   23
DEAN, JAMES   87, 203
DEATH CERTIFICATE   15, 46
DEATH PENALTY   116–117, 118
DEBILITY   106
DECAPITATIONS   123
DECATUR, STEPHEN   190
DEFECTIVE EQUIPMENT   81
DEFINITION OF DEATH   8
DEMOCRATS   16, 128, 132
DIABETES   214
DIAMOND, "LEGS"   208
DICKENS, CHARLES   195
DICKINSON, EMILY   193
DIDEROT   199
DILLINGER, JOHN   198
DISASTERS   67, 80, 83, 161
DISEASES   19, 22–25, 33, 35–37, 42,
   44–49, 52, 135–137

DISEMBOWLMENT 98
DISMEMBERING 121
DIVORCE RATE 91, 213
DOCTORS 15, 52–53
DOGS 45, 179
DOMESTIC ANIMALS 24
DOMINIS, ANTONIO 129
DOSTOYEVSKY, FYODOR 186
DOUGLASS, FREDERICK 186
DRAWBRIDGES 81
DRESDEN, ATTACK ON 187
DREW, DR. CHARLES 190
DRINKING 101
DROUGHT 19
DROWNINGS 58, 59, 67, 101
DRUG ABUSE 92, 102
DRUG OVERDOSES 18, 89, 100, 101,
   103
DRUG-INFLUENCED MURDERS 114
DRUGS 13, 18, 50
DRUNK DRIVERS 74, 78
DRUZE MOSLEMS 158
DUKE OF MONMOUTH 124
DUKE OF WINDSOR 194
DUNCAN, ISADORA 202
DUST 35, 66
DYNAMITE 65
DYSENTERY 49, 135
DYSPEPSIA 106

EARL OF ESSEX 123
EARTH FISSURES 171, 172
EARTHQUAKES 171–172
EDDY, MARY BAKER 208
EDISON, THOMAS ALVA 204
EDITORIAL HAZARDS 129
EICHMANN, ADOLF 194
EINSTEIN, ALBERT 192
EISENHOWER, DWIGHT D. 190
ELDERLY 36, 38, 91, 92, 96
ELECTRIC CHAIR 120
ELECTRIC EELS 181
ELECTROCUTION 133
ELIOT, T.S. 184
ELLIOT, CASS 199
EMERGENCY VEHICLES 72
EMOTIONAL CYCLE 17, 18
EMPEROR CONSTANTINE 125
EMPHYSEMA 9
ENGLAND 10, 11, 23, 50, 53, 68, 69, 70
EPIDEMICS 11, 30, 35, 43, 45, 46,
   47–49
EPILEPSY 106
EPSTEIN, BRIAN 89, 201
EQUIPMENT ACCIDENTS 64
ERRORS 52, 53
EUTHANASIA 116
EVERS, MEDGAR 115
EVOLUTION 43, 48

EXAMINATIONS 52
EXECUTIONS 108, 113, 116, 117, 121,
   123, 126
EXORCISM 197
EXPLOSIONS 64, 65, 66
EXPLOSIVES 95, 99, 141

FAINTING 69
FAIRBANKS, CHARLES W. 195
FALLS 58
FAMINE 19, 20, 21, 23
FAMOUS PEOPLE 87, 89, 102
FARMING 20, 64, 72
FAROUK I 189
FATAL ARGUMENTS 111
FEDERAL GOVERNMENT 40
FELONIES 111
FEMALE SUICIDE RATES 93
FEVERS 22
FIELDS, W.C. 209
FILARIASIS 24
FILLMORE, MILLARD 188
FINCH, PETER 185
FIRE 58, 59, 61–63
FIREARMS 89, 90, 92, 95, 100, 109, 112
FIREFIGHTER DEATHS 62
FIREPOWER 140
FISHER, JOHN 130
FITZGERALD, ZELDA SAYRE 189
FLEAS 44
FLIESS, WILHELM 17
FLOGGING 121
FLOODING 19, 173
FLOYD, "PRETTY BOY" 204
FLU 30, 34, 35, 44, 46
FLYING 80, 82–83
FOG 79, 169
FOOD 25, 30, 32, 44
FORRESTAL, JAMES 194
FOSTER, STEPHEN 185
FRANCO, FRANCISCO 207
FRANCO-GERMAN 143
FRANK, LEO 200
FRANKLIN, BENJAMIN 191
FREED, ALAN 185
FREUD, SIGMUND 17, 203
FRISCHLIN, NICODEMUS 131
FULTON, ROBERT 188
FUNERAL DIRECTORS 15

GABLE, CLARK 18
GAJDUSEK, DR
GALILEI, GALILEO 184
GANDHI, INDIRA 159
GARDNER, ERLE STANLEY 189
GARFIELD, JAMES 115, 203
GARFIELD, JOHN 194
GARGARIN, YURI 190

GARLAND, JUDY 18, 89, 196
GARNER, JOHN NANCE 206
GARRETT, PAT 198
GAS PAINS 146
GAS WARFARE 146–149
GASOLINE 74, 75
GASSES 35, 58, 64
GASSING 58, 89, 147
GASTRITIS 43
GEHRIG, LOU 195
GELLER, MAX 113, 198
GENOCIDE 155
GENOVESE, KITTY 189
"GENTLEMAN JIM" 187
GERRY, ELBRIDGE 207
GERSHWIN, GEORGE 196
GIARDIASIS 24
GILA MONSTERS 178
GILBERT, W.S. 194
GILMORE, GARY 117, 185
GOEBEL, WILLIAM 115
GOERING, HERMANN 204
GOLDEN GATE BRIDGE 93, 174
GOLFING 164
GOODYEAR, CHARLES 197
GRAIN ELEVATORS 64
GRANDIER, URBAN 130
GRANT, ULYSSES S. 199
GREEK ORTHODOX CHRISTIANS 158
GREEKS 11, 97
GREELEY, HORACE 207
GREY, LADY JANE 123
GRISSOM, VIRGIL 186
GRIZZLY BEARS 180
GROUP PANIC 69
GUEVARA, CHE 204
GUILLOTINES 123

HAIL 165–166
HALE, NATHAN 203
HALEY, BILL 187
HAMILTON, ALEXANDER 198
HAMLIN, HANNIBAL 197
HAMMARSKJOLD, DAG 87
HAMPTON, FRED 208
HANDGUNS 109, 111, 112, 115
"HANGING" PARKER 201
HANGINGS 89, 90, 101, 116, 120, 121
HARDIN, JOHN WESLEY 201
HARDIN, TIM 89
HARDING, WARREN G. 199
HARDY, THOMAS 185
HARI, MATA 204
HARLOW, JEAN 195
HARRISON, BENJAMIN 189
HARRISON, CARTER 115, 205
HARRISON, WILLIAM HENRY 191
HATHAWAY, DONNY 185

HAYES, RUTHERFORD B. 185
HEAD-HUNTERS 25–26
HEALTH FACILITIES 10, 55
HEART 30, 31, 37, 212
HEART ATTACK 18, 20, 28, 30, 31, 54, 55, 62
HEART DISEASE 13, 26–32, 38, 56, 88, 101, 214
HEINE, HEINRICH 187
HELICOPTERS 83, 84
HEMINGWAY, ERNEST 89, 197
HENDRICKS, THOMAS ANDREWS 207
HENDRIX, JIMI 102, 202
HEPATITUS 214
HERETICS 157
HICKOCK, RICHARD 206
HICKOK, "WILD BILL" 199
HIGH BLOOD PRESSURE 28, 31
HINDUS 98, 158
HIPPOCRATES 22
HIROSHIMA 151, 152, 153, 200
HISTORICAL WAR FATALITIES 150
HITLER, ADOLF 193
HOBART, BARRET AUGUSTUS 207
HODGKIN'S DISEASE 40
HOLLIDAY, "DOC" 206
HOLLIDAY, BILLIE "LADY DAY" 197
HOLLY, BUDDY 87, 186
HOLY WARS 99, 157–159
HOME 56, 58, 60, 61, 71
HOMICIDE 13, 108–133, 213, 214
HOMICIDE AND MOON PHASES 174
HOMICIDE DEFINITIONS 108–109
HOOKWORM 24
HOOVER, HERBERT 204
HOOVER, J. EDGAR 193
"HOPALONG CASSIDY" 202
HORNETS 178
HORSES 45, 68, 70, 159
HORSESBACK RIDING 164
HOSPITALS 51, 52, 55
HOT TUBS 101
HOUSTON, SAM 199
HOWARD, CATHERINE 187
HUGHES, HOWARD 191
HUMAN COMBUSTION 176
HUMAN GUINEA PIGS 148, 120
HUMAN SACRIFICES 127
HURRICANES 167
HUXLEY, ALDOUS 207
HYPOTHERMIA 12–13, 136

ILLEGAL DRUGS 102, 103
ILLEGITIMATE OFFSPRING 125
IMMUNITY 43, 45, 46
IMMUNOTHERAPY 37
INDIA 19, 21, 50, 98, 124, 158, 182
INDUSTRY 9, 59, 64

INFANTS   11, 34, 41–42, 108, 124–126
INFANTICIDE   108, 124–126
INFECTIONS   43, 47, 214
INFECTIOUS DISEASES   32, 42–46,
   135
INFLUENZA   33–36, 43, 45, 46, 49, 135,
   214
INQUISITION   129, 130, 157
INSECTS   177
INSECTICIDES   23
INTERNATIONAL DEATH PENALTIES
   118
IRREVERSIBLE COMA   9
ISRAEL   60, 142, 158
IVAN THE TERRIBLE   189

JACKSON, ANDREW   195
JACKSON, GENERAL "STONEWALL"
   193
JACKSON, GEORGE   201
JACKSON, WILLIAM HENRY   192
JAGUARS   179
JAMES, JESSE   191
JAPAN   10, 41, 50, 59, 60, 69, 98, 182
JEEPS   79–80
JEFFERSON, THOMAS   16, 197
JEWS   97, 155, 158
JIHAD   99
JOHN L. AVERY
JOHN THE BAPTIST   123
JOHNSON, ANDREW   199
JOHNSON, LYNDON   185
JOHNSON, RICHARD MENTOR   207
JOLSON, AL   205
JONES, BRIAN   197
JONES, CASEY   80
JONES, DAVEY   87
JONES, JIM   89, 98, 206
JOPLIN, JANIS   18, 102, 203
JOPLIN, SCOTT   190
JUSTIFIABLE HOMICIDE   109

KAMIKAZE BOMBERS   98
KATH, TERRY   185
KEATON, BUSTER   186
KELLER, HELEN   195
KELLY, GRACE   87
KEMMLER, WILLIAM   120, 200
KENNEDY, EDWARD   198
KENNEDY, JOHN F.   115, 207
KENNEDY, PATRICK BOUVIER   200
KENNEDY, ROBERT   116, 195
KERN, JEROME   206
KETCHUM, "BLACK JACK"   192
KHAN, GENGHIS   45, 200
KIDD, CAPTAIN WILLIAM   194
KIDNEYS   40, 214
KING, ALBERTA   196

KING, REVEREND MARTIN LUTHER
   116
KING, WILLIAM RUFUS DE VANE   191
KNOW-NOTHING PARTY   132
KOMAROV, VLADIMIR   192
KOPECHNE, MARY JO   198
KURU   25

LANDIS, CAROLE   89
LANDSLIDES   169
LAVA   170
"LAWRENCE OF ARABIA"   194
LAZARUS   208
LEE, BRUCE   198
LEE, GYPSY ROSE   192
LEE, ROBERT E.   204
LEGAL DRUGS   102
LEGAL INSTITUTIONS   8
LEGAL INTERVENTION   101, 108, 214
LEISHMANIASIS   24
LEOPARDS   179
LEUKEMIA   40
LEWIS, SINCLAIR   184
LIFE EXPECTANCIES   10, 11, 12, 27,
   32, 38, 50
LIFE SPANS   10, 11
LIGHTNING   111, 162–165
LINCOLN, ABRAHAM   115, 191
LIONS   179
LIQUID GAS   65
LISTER, JOSEPH   51, 187
LITTLE MERMAID   124
LIVE BIRTHS   42
LIVER   214
LOCKHART, FRANK   192
LOMBARD, CAROLE   87, 185
LONDON, JACK   102
LONG, HUEY P.   115
LONGEVITY   42, 50
LONGFELLOW, HENRY WADSWORTH
   190
LOUIS XVI   124, 185
LUNAR THEORIES   173
LUNG   40
LUNG CANCER   38, 39
LUTHER, MARTIN   197
LYMON, FRANKIE   188
LYNCH, CAPTAIN WILLIAM   120
LYNCH, JUDGE CHARLES   121
LYNCHING   120–123

MADERO, FRANCISCO   174
MADISON, JAMES   196
MALARIA   22–23, 24, 45, 49
MALCOLM X   115, 188
MALIGNANCIES   214
MALNUTRITION   20, 136
MANILA BAY, BATTLE OF   193

MANSFIELD, JAYNE 87, 196
MANSFIELD, KATHERINE 184
MANSLAUGHTER 89, 108
MANSON, CHARLES 200
MARAT, JEAN PAUL 198
MARCIANO, ROCKY 87, 201
MARCUS SALVIUS OTHO 191
MARINES 79, 80, 138
MARKSMANSHIP 141
MARLEY, BOB 193
MARLOWE, CHRISTOPHER 89
MARSHALL, THOMAS RILEY 195
MARX, KARL 189
MARY, QUEEN OF SCOTS 123
MASS MURDER 134
MASS TRANSPORTATION 82
MASTURBATION 106
MATERNAL DEATHS 41, 53
MATRICIDE 109
MAUPASSANT, GUY DE 197
MCALLISTER, BILLY JOE 195
MCKINLEY, WILLIAM 18, 115, 202
MEASLES 45, 49
MEDICAL STUDENTS 53
MEDITERRANEAN 23, 48
MEIN, JOHN GORDON 201
MELVILLE, HERMAN 177
MENINGITIS 35, 214
MENTAL PATIENTS 92
MICHEL, ANNELIESE 197
MICROORGANISMS 42, 43, 44, 45
MICROWAVE RADIATION 29
MIDDLE AGES 98, 126, 157
MILITARY EXECUTIONS 117
MILITARY FATALITIES 80, 138, 139,
　145, 150
MILITARY INVASIONS 45, 46
MILLER, GLEN 87
MILLS, LUCINDA 187
MILNE, A.A. 186
MINEO, SAL 187
MINING 35, 59, 66
MICROWAVES 28
MISS FITZSIMMONS 195
MISSILES 142
MITCHELL, MARGARET 87, 200
MOBS 120, 132
MOLINA, RAFAEL TRUJILLO 174
MOLLUSKS 181
MOLLY MCGUIRES 196
MONROE, JAMES 197
MONROE, MARILYN 18, 89, 102, 200
MOON PHASES 173
MOON, KEITH 102
MOORE, GEORGE C. 116
MORE, SIR THOMAS 124
MORMONS 158
MORRISON, JIM 197
MORRISON, NORMAN 205
MORTON, LEVI PARSONS 194

MOSLEMS 48, 88, 97, 157
MOSQUITOS 22, 23
MOTOR VEHICLE ACCIDENTS 56, 59,
　70, 71, 74, 78
MOTORCYCLES 72
MOUNTAIN LIONS 179
MOZART, WOLFGANG AMADEUS
　208
MUNI, PAUL 201
MUNITIONS 65, 140, 142
MUNSON, THURMAN 87, 199
MURDER 14, 15, 54, 89–133
MURPHY, AUDIE 87
MUSSOLINI, BENITO 192
MUSTARD GAS 146, 149
MYOCARDIAL INFARCTION 30

NAGASAKI 151, 152, 153, 200
NASSER, GAMAL ABDEL 203
NATION, CARRY 195
NATIONALIST FANATICS 98
NATURAL DISASTERS 19, 161
NATURAL GAS 65
NATURAL KILLERS 160–183
NAVY 29, 79, 80, 138, 139
NAZIS 156
NEANDERTHAL MAN 11
NEHRU, JAWAHARLAL 194
NELSON, ADMIRAL HORATIO 204
NELSON, GEORGE "BABY FACE" 207
NEO-NATAL 53
NEOLITHIC REVOLUTION 19
NEOPLASMS 214
NERO 89
NERVE GASES 147
NEUROBLASTOMA 40
NEWBORN 124
NIGHTINGALE, FLORENCE 136
NOEL, CLEO A. 116
NOISE DEATHS 54–55
NON-COMBAT FATALITIES 135, 138
NURSING 136
NURSING HOMES 55

OBESITY 32
OCEAN TRAVEL 86, 87
OCHS, PHIL 191
ONCHOCERCIASIS 24
OPEN BRIDGES 81
OPERATIONS 51
OSWALD, LEE HARVEY 184
OVARIES 40
OVERDOSES 15, 18, 89, 103
OVEREXPOSURE 12

PACKER, ALFERD 128
PAINE, THOMAS 195

PALEARIUS, ANTONIUS   130
PANICS   69
PARALYSIS   31
PARASITES   22, 23–24, 42, 43, 46
PARKER, CHARLIE   189
PASSENGERS   70, 72, 76, 77, 82, 84, 86
PASTEUR, LOUIS   42
PATHOLOGISTS   14
PATIENTS   37, 38, 39, 52, 62
PATRICIDE108
PATTON, GEORGE   87, 209
PAVLOV, IVAN   188
PAVLOVA, ANNA   186
PEDESTRIANS   75
PERINATAL CONDITIONS   214
PERSECUTIONS   155–156
PETIT, PIERRE   131
PHENOTHIAZINES   13
PHOSGENE GAS   146
PHYSICIAN RATIO   213
PICASSO, PABLO   191
PICNICKING   164
PIERCE, FRANKLIN   204
PIGS   24, 44, 45
PILOT THE DOG   204
PINKERTON, ALLAN   197
PIRANHAS   180
PITT, WILLIAM   185
THE PLAGUE   47, 149
PLAGUES   19, 47, 49, 149
PLANES   70, 81, 84
PLATO   97
PLINY THE ELDER   201
PNEUMONIA   9, 33, 34, 35, 36, 43, 46,
    101, 214
POCAHONTAS   190
POE, EDGAR ALLEN   203
POGRAMS   156
POISONS   58, 59, 89, 90, 95
POISON GAS   146
POISONOUS ANIMALS   177–178
POISONOUS FUMES   169
POLAR BEARS   180
POLICEMEN   92
POLITICAL CONFLICTS   20
POLITICAL UNREST   132
POLK, JAMES KNOX   196
POLLACK, JACKSON   87, 200
POLLUTION   9, 169
POMPEY THE GREAT   203
POPULATION   19, 25, 27, 34, 36, 38, 41,
    44, 45, 46, 71, 75, 125, 213
PORTUGUESE MAN-OF-WAR   178
POST, WILEY   200
POWERS, FRANCIS GARY   83
PRESCRIBED DRUGS   102
PRESIDENTS   16
PRESLEY, ELVIS   200
PRINCE FAISAL   124
PRINCE MUSEID   196

PRINZE, FREDDIE   186
PRISONERS OF WAR   148, 153
PROGNOSIS   37
PROHIBITION   105
PROSTATE   40, 214
PROSTITUTION   125
PROTESTANTS   157
PUBLIC EXECUTIONS   117
PUBLIC LYNCHING   121
PULMONARY DEATHS   212
PURVIS, MELVIN   188
PYLE, ERNIE   191
PYTHAGORAS   97

QUAKERS   158
QUEEN ASTRID   201

RABIES   44
RACE   34, 35, 118, 120, 122, 133
RADIATION   28, 66, 152
RAILROAD TRAINS   68, 70, 78, 80–81,
    82
RALEIGH, SIR WALTER   124
RASPUTIN, GRIGORI   208
RATTLESNAKES   177
RECTUM   40
REDDING, OTIS   87, 208
"REDLIGHT BANDIT"   193
REINKING, THEODORE   131
RELIGIOUS FANATICS   98
RELIGIOUS PERSECUTIONS
    157–159
RELIGIOUS PILGRIMMAGES   46
RELIGIOUS RITES   127
RELIGIOUS SACRIFICES   124
REPUBLICANS   16, 128
RESEARCH   24, 25, 26, 52, 55, 147
RESPIRATION   9
RESPIRATORY DISESASES   9
REVERE, PAUL   193
RHEUMATIC FEVER   31
RHEUMATIC HEART DISEASE   28, 31
RICKETS   106
RIN TIN TIN   200
RINDERPEST   44
RINDFLEISCH MASSACRE   155
RINGLING BROTHERS CIRCUS   197
RIOTS   132–133, 157
RITUALS   25, 26, 98
RIVERS   87, 173
ROBESPIERRE, MAXIMILIAN   124
ROCK SLIDES   168, 169
ROCKEFELLER, NELSON   186
ROCKETS   141, 142
ROCKNE, KNUTE   87
ROCKWELL, GEORGE LINCOLN   201
RODENTS   44
ROEBLING, JOHN   198

ROGERS, WILL 87, 200
ROMANS 11, 23, 47, 48, 97, 98
ROMANTIC TRIANGLES 111
ROMEO AND JULIET 89
ROOSEVELT, ELEANOR 206
ROOSEVELT, FRANKLIN D. 133, 189, 191
ROOSEVELT, THEODORE 184
ROTHKO, MARK 188
ROUNDWORM 24
RUBY, JACK 184
RUSSELL, BERTRAND 186
RUSSIA 21, 83, 156
RUTH, GEORGE HERMAN "BABE" 200
RYAN, REP. LEO 207

SACCO, NICOLA 201
SADAT, ANWAR 203
SAFETY 66, 68, 69, 70, 73, 76, 83, 86
SAILORS 87, 128
SAINT ALBAN 123
SAINT BERNADETTE 191
SAINT FRANCIS OF ASSISI 203
SAINT GEORGE 123
SAINT PAUL 123
SAINT THOMAS AQUINAS 188
SAMSON 89, 97
SAN QUENTIN PRISON 99, 193, 201
SANITATION 46, 51, 135
SATAN 98
SATTEE 98
SAUL 89, 97
SAX, ADOLPHE 187
SCHUBERT, FRANZ 207
SCHWEITZER, ALBERT 201
SCORPIONS 177
SCRIPPS, EDWARD 189
SCUBA DIVERS 183
SEA LIONS 183
SEE, ELLIOT 188
SELF-DEFENSE 109
SELF-IMMOLATION 101
SELF-STRANGULATION 107
SELFRIDGE, THOMAS 202
SEPEKU 98
SEPTICEMIA 214
SEWAGE 44
SEX OFFENSES 111
SHAFFER, COL. PAUL R. SHAFFER 116
SHAKESPEARE, WILLIAM 192
SHARKS 182–183
SHAW, GEORGE BERNARD 205
SHERMAN, JAMES SCHOOLCRAFT 205
SHIITE MOSLEMS 99, 158
SHIPS 86–87
SIDNEY, ALGERNON 130

SIEGEL, "BUGSY" 196
SIKHS 158
SILICOSIS 66
SINATRA, DOLLY 87
SITTING BULL 208
SMALLPOX 44, 45, 48, 49
SMITH, JOSEPH 196
SMITH, PERRY 206
SMOKE INHALATION 62
SMOKING 28, 32, 61
SNAKE BITES 177, 181–182
SNAKE SERUM FATALITIES 178
SNOW 79, 168, 169
SOAP OPERA SUICIDES 96
SOCRATES 89
SOLDIERS 68, 92, 135
SOUSA, JOHN PHILIP 188
SPAS 101
SPECK, RICHARD 198
SPEED LIMIT 56, 70, 71, 75, 76, 66, 80
SPIDERS 177
SPONTANEOUS COMBUSTION 176–177
SRI LANKA 159
STABBINGS 112
STARR, BELLE 186
STARVATION 19–21
STATE RANKINGS 212–213
STATE SUICIDE RATES 91
STATUTORY DEATH PENALTIES 117
STEINBECK, JOHN 209
STEVENSON, ADLAI 198
STEVENSON, ADLAI EWING 196
STINGRAYS 181
STOMACH CANCER 40
STOWE, HARRIET BEECHER 197
STRANGULATIONS 90, 107, 112
STRAVINSKY, IGOR 191
STREPTOCOCCAL INFECTION 31
STRESS 32
STROKES 13, 28, 31, 32–33, 55, 56, 212, 213
STRUCTURAL FAILURES 67
STRUCTURE FIRES 63
SUBMARINES 144
SUICIDES 13, 14, 15, 54, 88–107, 125, 174, 212, 214
SULLIVAN, ROY 111
SUNNI MOSLEMS 158
SURGERY 51
SURVIVAL 37, 38, 40, 52, 70, 127, 162
SWEATING SICKNESS 49
SWEDEN 10, 27, 50, 60
SYMBIONESE LIBERATION ARMY 194

TAFT, WILLIAM H. 188
TAMILS 159
TATE, SHARON 200
TAXIS 72

TAYLOR, ZACHARY   198
TB (SEE TUBERCULOSIS)
TEACH, EDWARD   207
TEACHING HOSPITALS   53
TELEVISION   21, 83, 91, 96
TERRORISM   85, 98
TESLA, NICOLA   184
TESTES   40
TETANUS   149
"THE BIG BOPPER"   87
"THE HIGHWAYMAN"   191
THOMAS, DYLAN   102
THOREAU, HENRY DAVID   193
THUCYDIDES   47
THUMB, TOM   184
THUNDERSTORMS   162, 163, 165
TICKS   178
TIGERS   179
TODD, MICHAEL   87, 190
TOMPKINS, DANIEL D.   195
TORNADOS   166-167
TORPEDOS   144
TRAFFIC ACCIDENTS   18, 56, 68, 71,
    72, 74, 79
TRAINS (SEE RAILROAD TRAINS)
TRANSPORTATION ACCIDENTS   59,
    65, 70-87, 138
TRICHURIASIS   24
TROTSKY, LEON   174, 201
TRUMAN, HARRY   209
TRYPANOSOMIASIS   24
TSE-TUNG, MAO   202
TUBERCULOSIS   36, 43, 135, 214
TUBMAN, HARRIET   189
TURKISH MOSLEMS   158
TURNER, LT. COL. JOHN H.   116
TURNPIKES   73
TURPIN, RICHARD   191
TWAIN, MARK   192
TWISTERS (SEE TORNADOS)
TYLER, JOHN   185
TYPHOID   135, 149
TYPHOID MARY   206
TYPHUS   45, 49

UPHOLSTERY FIRES   61
URANIUM   66
UTERUS   40

VACCINES   23, 42
VALENS, RITCHIE   186
VALENTINO, RUDOLPH   201
VALIUM   13
VANINI, LUCILIO   130
VANZETTI, BARTOLOMEO   201
VENDETTAS   113
VERNE, JULES   190
VICE PRESIDENTS   16

VICIOUS, SID   186
VICTIMS   35, 38, 62
VIGILANTE JUSTICE   120
VILLA, PANCHO   188
VIRAL AGENTS   46
VIRUS   25
VOLCANOS   170

WADLOW, ROBERT   198
WAGNER, DR. HAL   14-15
WALLACE, HENRY A.   206
WALLENDA, KARL   190
WARS   19, 71, 91, 134-159, 210-211
WARREN, LEONARD   188
WASHINGTON, GEORGE   208
WASHKANSKY, LOUIS   209
WASPS   177
WATER ACTIVITIES   164
WATER MOCCASINS   178
WEAPONS   48, 112
WEATHER   19, 78, 79, 83
WEISER, CASPAR   131
WEISSMULLER, JOHNNY   185
WET NURSES   126
WHEELER, WILLIAM ALMON   195
WHIGS   132
WHITE, EDWARD   186
WHITMAN, CHARLES   199
WHITMAN, WALT   190
WILLIAM KOGUT   99
WILLIAMS, HANK   184
WILLIAMS, JOHN   131
WILLIAMS, WILLIAM CARLOS   188
WILSON, HENRY   207
WILSON, WOODROW   186
WIRZ, HENRY   206
WITCHES   157
WOLVES   179
WOOLF, VIRGINIA   89, 190
WORK   58, 59, 60, 64, 65, 66
WRIGHT, ORVILLE   186
WRITERS   129

YABLONSKI, JOSEPH   184
YELLOW FEVER   49
YELLOWJACKETS   177

ZANGARA, GUISEPPE   133, 189
"ZIPPY THE PINHEAD"   192
ZULUS   185